"The intersection of the computational, biological, and medical sciences is poised to revolutionize personalized medicine across a vast spectrum of diseases and in low-, medium-, and high-income countries. This new book, *Data Driven Science for Clinically Actionable Knowledge in Diseases*, serves as a fantastic overview of the space for all stakeholders. The text enables readers to learn both about the trajectory of the space and to identify specific technical use cases where success has been shown and which can be re-deployed into new systems."
—**Dr Noah Berlow,** *First Ascent Biomedical*

"Health data is inherently complex and collected via wildly diverse channels. This book shows how leveraging health data is difficult, difficult to collect, and difficult to synthesise, but how much patient care can be improved when it is done well."
—**Prof David Skillicorn,** *Queens University, Kingston, Ontario, Canada*

Data Driven Science for Clinically Actionable Knowledge in Diseases

Data-driven science has become a major decision-making aid for the diagnosis and treatment of disease. Computational and visual analytics enables effective exploration and sense making of large and complex data through the deployment of appropriate data science methods, meaningful visualisation and human-information interaction.

This edited volume covers state-of-the-art theory, method, models, design, evaluation and applications in computational and visual analytics in desktop, mobile and immersive environments for analysing biomedical and health data. The book is focused on data-driven integral analysis, including computational methods and visual analytics practices and solutions for discovering actionable knowledge in support of clinical actions in real environments.

By studying how data and visual analytics have been implemented into the healthcare domain, the book demonstrates how analytics influences the domain through improving decision making, specifying diagnostics, selecting the best treatments and generating clinical certainty.

Daniel R. Catchpoole is the Group Leader of the Tumour Bank, Children's Cancer Research Unit, Children's Hospital, Westmead, Australia. He is also affiliated with the Faculty of Medicine at the University of Sydney and the Department of Information Technology at the University of Technology Sydney.

Simeon J. Simoff is the Cluster Pro Vice Chancellor (Science, Technology, Engineering and Mathematics) and Dean of the School of Computer, Data and Mathematical Sciences at Western Sydney University.

Paul J. Kennedy is the Director of the Biomedical Data Science Laboratory at the Australia Artificial Intelligence Institute and the Head of Computer Science in the Faculty of Engineering and Information Technology at the University of Technology Sydney.

Quang Vinh Nguyen is the Director of Academic Programs for Postgraduate ICT at the School of Computer, Data and Mathematical Sciences and the MARCS Institute for Brain, Behaviour and Development at Western Sydney University.

Analytics and AI for Healthcare

Artificial Intelligence (AI) and analytics are increasingly being applied to various healthcare settings. AI and analytics are salient to facilitate better understanding and identifying key insights from healthcare data in many areas of practice and enquiry including at the genomic, individual, hospital, community and/ or population levels. The Chapman & Hall/CRC Press Analytics and AI in Healthcare Series aims to help professionals upskill and leverage the techniques, tools, technologies and tactics of analytics and AI to achieve better healthcare delivery, access, and outcomes. The series covers all areas of analytics and AI as applied to healthcare. It will look at critical areas including prevention, prediction, diagnosis, treatment, monitoring, rehabilitation and survivorship.

About the Series Editor

Professor Nilmini Wickramasinghe is Professor of Digital Health and the Deputy Director of the Iverson Health Innovation Research Institute at Swinburne University of Technology, Australia and is inaugural Professor—Director Health Informatics Management at Epworth HealthCare, Victoria, Australia. She also holds honorary research professor positions at the Peter MacCallum Cancer Centre, Murdoch Children's Research Institute and Northern Health. For over 20 years, Professor Wickramasinghe has been researching and teaching within the health informatics/digital health domain. She was awarded the prestigious Alexander von Humboldt award in recognition of her outstanding contribution to digital health.

Explainable AI in Healthcare
Edited by Mehul S Raval, Mohendra Roy, Tolga Kaya, and Rupal Kapdi

Data Analysis in Medicine and Health Using R
Kamarul Imran Musa, Wan Nor Arifin Wan Mansor, and Tengku Muhammad Hanis

Data Driven Science for Clinically Actionable Knowledge in Diseases
Edited by Daniel R. Catchpoole, Simeon J. Simoff, Paul J. Kennedy, and Quang Vinh Nguyen

For more information about this series please visit: www.routledge.com/ analytics-and-ai-for-healthcare/book-series/Aforhealth

Data Driven Science for Clinically Actionable Knowledge in Diseases

Edited by
Daniel R. Catchpoole
Simeon J. Simoff
Paul J. Kennedy
Quang Vinh Nguyen

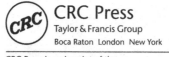

CRC Press
Taylor & Francis Group
Boca Raton London New York

CRC Press is an imprint of the
Taylor & Francis Group, an **informa** business
A CHAPMAN & HALL BOOK

Designed cover image: A 3D rendering of an abstract technology group and social network connection on a blurry background

First edition published 2024
by CRC Press
2385 NW Executive Center Drive, Suite 320, Boca Raton FL 33431

and by CRC Press
4 Park Square, Milton Park, Abingdon, Oxon, OX14 4RN

CRC Press is an imprint of Taylor & Francis Group, LLC

ISBN: 978-1-032-27353-2 (hbk)
ISBN: 978-1-032-27351-8 (pbk)
ISBN: 978-1-003-29235-7 (ebk)

DOI: 10.1201/9781003292357

Typeset in Minion Pro
by Apex CoVantage, LLC

Contents

Contributors

Ilias Aitterrami received his Master of Science at the Department of Statistics and Applied Probability, National University of Singapore. He is working as a project engineer at Nexans.

Professor **Daniel R. Catchpoole** is Group Leader of the Tumour Bank, Children's Cancer Research Unit at the Children's Hospital at Westmead, Australia. He is also affiliated with the Faculty of Medicine at the University of Sydney and of Information Technology at the University of Technology Sydney.

Dr **Avijit Kumar Chaudhuri** is an assistant professor in the Department of Computer Science and Engineering, Techno Engineering College Banipur, Kolkata, India.

Tanzila K. Chowdhury is a PhD candidate at the Centre for Research in Mathematics and Data Science, Western Sydney University. She is a senior research and evaluation analyst at CESE, NSW Department of Education.

Dr **Allison Clarke** is Director of the External Data Partnerships and Capability Section, Health Economics and Research Division, Australian Department of Health. She has worked across Medicare, hospitals and data analytic areas and has a sound understanding of government health programs and priorities at both the state and national levels.

Patricia Correll is a principal epidemiologist of the NSW Ministry of Health with the NSW Ministry of Health. The author has contributed to research in topics of population and public health informatics.

Jamil Daher received his tertiary education in computer science at the School of Computer Science, University of Technology Sydney. He is working as data engineer at Macquarie Group.

Professor **Barry Drake** is an industry professor in the School of Computer Science at the University of Technology Sydney. Barry's research is directed towards algorithms and software for making practical smart systems, with a focus on fast, efficient, accurate methods.

Professor **Edouard Duchesnay** is a research director in machine learning applied to neuroimaging at NeuroSpin, CEA, Paris-Saclay, France. He supervises the design of machine learning and statistical models to uncover neural signatures predictive of clinical trajectories in psychiatric disorders.

Marc Fischer is with the Institute of Signal Processing and System Theory, University of Stuttgart, Germany.

Professor **Andrew Francis** is the Deputy Dean of the School of Computer, Data, and Mathematical Sciences, Western Sydney University. He is a former ARC Future Fellow who works on a wide range of research problems in algebra and mathematical biology.

Associate Professor **Carol Anne Hargreaves** is the Director of the Data Analytics Consulting Centre, Department of Statistics and Data Science, Department of Mathematics, Faculty of Science, National University of Singapore.

Girija Rani Karetla is a PhD candidate in the School of Computer, Data and Mathematical Sciences, Western Sydney University. Her research focuses on deep neural networks for classification of biomedical data.

Professor **Paul J. Kennedy** is the Director of the Biomedical Data Science Laboratory at the Australia Artificial Intelligence Institute and Head of Computer Science in the Faculty of Engineering and Information Technology at the University of Technology Sydney.

Chng Wei Lau is a PhD candidate in the School of Computer, Data and Mathematical Sciences, Western Sydney University. His research focuses on immersive analytics for oncology patient cohorts, machine learning and visualisation.

Nico Loesch is a PhD student in the School of Computer Science at the University of Technology Sydney, Australia. His main research interest is applied artificial intelligence research applied to medical images.

Associate Professor **Guodong Long** joined the University of Technology Sydney (UTS) in 2010 and earned a PhD at UTS in 2014. His current research interest focuses on using federated learning to develop a trust-worthy AI with privacy-preserving and personalised intelligence.

Associate Professor **Quang Vinh Nguyen** is the Director of Academic Programs for Postgraduate ICT at the School of Computer, Data and Mathematical Sciences and the MARCS Institute for Brain, Behaviour and Development at Western Sydney University.

Associate Professor **Laurence A.F. Park** is the Director of Academic Programs—Data Science, Centre for Research in Mathematics and Data Science, School of Computer, Data and Mathematical Sciences, Western Sydney University, Australia. He is currently investigating methods of large-scale data mining and machine learning.

Dr. **Xueping Peng** is a lecturer at the Australian Artificial Intelligence Institute (AAII), University of Technology Sydney, Australia. He earned a dual PhD at UTS in 2015 and the Beijing Institute of Technology (China) in 2013.

Zhonglin Qu is a PhD candidate in the School of Computer, Data and Mathematical Sciences, Western Sydney University. Her research focuses on explainable artificial intelligence and interpretability of biomedical data.

Arkadip Ray is with the Department of Information Technology, Government College of Engineering and Ceramic Technology, Kolkata, India.

Professor **Simeon J. Simoff** is Cluster Pro Vice Chancellor (Science, Technology, Engineering and Mathematics) and Dean of the School of Computer, Data and Mathematical Sciences at Western Sydney University.

Professor **Glenn Stone** is with Insurance Australia Group Limited and an adjunct professor of Data Science at the School of Computer, Data and Mathematical Sciences. Dr Stone's interests are in computationally intensive methods with applications.

Professor **Mark M Tanaka** is a mathematical and computational biologist at the University of New South Wales (UNSW) in the School of Biotechnology and Biomolecular Sciences (BABS). He is also a member of the Evolution and Ecology Research Centre (E&ERC).

Wensi Tang is a PhD candidate at the Australian AI Institute, FEIT, University of Technology Sydney, Australia.

Yezihalem Tegegne is an MPhil candidate in the School of Computer, Data and Mathematical Sciences, Western Sydney University. His research focuses on optimisation of machine learning techniques for biomedical data.

Dr **Jesse Tran** is the founder of Gemtracks and a PhD graduate in computer science at the School of Computer, Data and Mathematical Sciences, Western Sydney University.

Peng Yan is a PhD candidate at the Australian AI Institute, FEIT, University of Technology Sydney, Australia.

Preface

0.1 DATA-DRIVEN SCIENCE FOR CLINICALLY ACTIONABLE KNOWLEDGE AND HEALTH POLICY

Data-driven science has become a major decision-making aid for public health policymakers, as well as the diagnosis and treatment of diseases. Computational and visual analytics enables effective exploration and makes sense of large and complex data through the deployment of appropriate data science methods, meaningful visualisation, and human–information interaction. This edited book covers state-of-the-art theories, technologies, methods, surveys, evaluations, guidelines, and applications for data-driven integral analysis in biomedical and health data. By studying how data and visual analytics have been implemented into the healthcare domain, we can demonstrate how analytics influences the domain by improving decision-making, specifying diagnostics, selecting the best treatments, and generating clinical certainty.

The book tackles important issues in personalised medicine and evidence-based decision-making that focuses on 'close the loop' analytical processes to enrich and lead actionable knowledge. By utilising inter- and transdisciplinary expertise and knowledge in computational and visual analytics, it enables better and more effective ways to engineer and discover actionable knowledge and knowledge representation schemata. The book also focuses on rare diseases where there are limited numbers of available samples and which cannot be handled effectively by ordinary methods and approaches.

The book suits a wide range of research students, tertiary students, and PhD candidates, as well as researchers in computing, data science, healthcare, and biology fields. The book is also useful to current medical practitioners or medical data analysts who are looking for data analytics methods and technologies and how analytics influences the health domain.

The book is aimed to be used by researchers and data analytics professionals in fields who are using current and new ideas and strategies for biomedical data analytics to gain insights into their data to support better personalised treatments. The book uniquely looks at the deep fusion of data-driven methods into health informatics that impact clinical care and health policymaking.

0.2 BOOK STRUCTURE

The book is organised into three sections. Section one (Chapter 1 to Chapter 3) covers studies on data-driven science for population health, including diabetes cohorts, the COVID-19 pandemic, and drug resistance of tuberculosis. Section two (Chapter 4 to Chapter 7) presents state-of-the-art computational analytic methods, models, and systems that enable effective ways to analyse large biomedical and health data. Section three (Chapter 8 to Chapter 10) focuses on the visual and human factors of the analytical processes, especially in interpretability and trust aspects. The chapters are summarised as follows.

0.2.1 Employing Data-Driven Science in Healthcare Studies

Chapter 1 presents an interesting study on the association between events in primary care and health outcomes with a large cohort of diabetes patients from the Lumis program of administrative health records from New South Wales, Australia, for the period of 2011 to 2020. This study utilised linked patient data to investigate the impact of patient journey patterns on health outcomes for patients with diabetes. The study identified several aspects of a patient's engagement with general practice (GP) services that were associated with either an improvement or worsening of health outcomes, including the timing of the first antidiabetic prescription, the presence of a management plan or health assessment, and telehealth usage. The authors carried out both univariate and multivariate analyses on several primary care events, including first antidiabetic prescription, health assessments, and general practice management plans. These findings provide guidance to GPs and governments on how healthcare delivery can be improved, particularly for high-risk patients. The study also highlights the usefulness of linked patient records for generating clinically actionable knowledge.

The COVID-19 pandemic has caused significant disruptions in healthcare delivery and had a profound impact on vulnerable populations, particularly patients with complex health conditions. Chapter 2 presents a literature review that provides valuable insights into how the pandemic has affected three specific cohorts of vulnerable populations: patients with chronic disease, patients with cancer, and patients with end-of-life care. The review highlights the need for data-driven analysis to inform policy decisions and improve the quality of life for these patients. The proposed analysis methodology and cancer-code mapping table can be useful tools for identifying vulnerable populations and developing targeted interventions. Ultimately, this review can help inform national response strategies for future pandemics and support clinical decision-making for the diagnosis and treatment of diseases in real-world environments

The increasing prevalence of drug-resistant tuberculosis (TB) is a significant public health concern, and understanding the relative contribution of transmission and treatment failure to this issue is critical for developing effective control strategies. Chapter 3 contributes an efficient computational method coupled with a graph visualisation to support the estimation of the relative contributions of transmission and treatment failure to the spread of drug resistance of tuberculosis. The method provides timely insights into the spread of drug-resistant TB, facilitating better decision-making for public health authorities. The next logical step is to expand the analysis to include multiple drug resistance and consider all possible paths towards cluster formation. These efforts will further enhance our understanding of the spread of drug-resistant TB and support effective disease control.

0.2.2 Computational Analytic Methods for Healthcare Derived Data

Chapter 4 introduces a novel diagnosis system for Parkinson's disease (PD) using an ensemble random forest model. PD is a leading cause of mortality globally, and diagnosing it accurately can be challenging for medical experts due to variations in test results. The proposed study aims to develop a PD prediction model using an ensemble random forest (ERF) classifier, which combines various classification approaches to improve accuracy. The study compared ERF with state-of-the-art classifiers, comparing the existing support vector machines, radial basis kernel, decision tree, and random forest. The results showed that ERF outperformed them all, achieving 96% accuracy and lower false positive/negative rates. The proposed ERF model can help medical practitioners in accurately diagnosing PD, particularly in low-income and middle-income countries, and improve patient outcomes

The increasing amount of brain data collected in recent years has led to a challenge in the harmonisation of the data across different sites and scanners due to inter-site variability. Chapter 5 presents a robust harmonisation method that was developed to remove this variability while preserving variability in brain MRI image data. The study used an adjusted linear regression model and a random effects model called ComBat to evaluate the harmonisation process but found that the ComBat method introduces bias when target information is introduced beforehand. Other methods to evaluate harmonisation without bias were explored, such as looking at the life-span trajectory of the data. The study concludes that, although visible, the bias did not have a huge impact on the evaluation of the models but poses a fundamental problem for the ComBat method in conforming to basic principles of machine learning.

Chapter 6 provides an overview and comparison of feature-ranking methods for a wide range of RNA sequencing datasets. RNA sequencing is a widely used technique for studying gene expression patterns, and feature-ranking methods have emerged as a powerful tool for analysing RNA sequencing data. This review describes different ways to rank features and how they can be used to gain insights into the underlying biology. The chapter compares state-of-the-art feature selection techniques, including machine learning techniques such as random forest, and discusses their advantages and limitations. The experimental findings suggest that random forest can be a better alternative for classifying large RNA-Seq datasets for biomedical research. However, studies may not manage feature redundancy or examine the impact of other characteristics, making it difficult to determine their relevance. Future directions for the development and use of feature-ranking techniques include the use of deep learning techniques, the use of single-cell sequencing data, and the development of methods for figuring out how genes interact with each other. The combination of both feature selection with feature-ranking processes can also improve the prediction outcomes in RNA sequencing data analytics.

Chapter 7 evaluates graph neural networks (GNNs) for brain tumour segmentation and their reformulation of feature aggregation for non-Euclidean data to assess glioma lesions in adults. The study compared three promising ConvGNNs and showed the potential spatial methods inherit over their spectral counterparts. The predominantly utilised GCN obtains insufficient segmentation results and is outperformed by GIN and GAT. The study also utilised the well-established U-Net architecture for semantic segmentation by combining both conventional and graph sub-networks. The full potential of graph operations is discussed, with analysis that enhances the precision and reliability of highly diffuse brain tumours.

0.2.3 Visualisation, Visual Analytics, and Human Factors

The emergence of biomedical data analytics has led to a significant impact on the diagnosis and treatment of diseases. Chapter 8 provides a comprehensive tutorial on the methods, technologies, and processes for biomedical data analysis. The chapter discusses computational analytics strategies such as feature selection, feature extraction, and clustering, along with various aspects of visual analytics and interactive visualisation, including emerging technologies such as virtual reality and augmented reality. The proposed framework provides a structured approach for researchers and students to study and develop methods in both computational and visual analytics, thus enabling the effective exploration and interpretation of complex biomedical data. This chapter serves as a guideline for biomedical data analysts to produce meaningful analytical outcomes and support decision-making in healthcare. In particular, it shows processes, computational analytics, visualisation, emerging technology, and case studies to illustrate the analytical work on such data.

The integration of machine learning and visualisation techniques in biomedical data analysis has become increasingly important in recent years. Chapter 9 discusses visualisation methods for interpreting supervised and unsupervised machine learning models and methods in the biomedical field. This chapter provides a comprehensive review of visualisation methods for explainable machine learning in biomedical data analysis. Visualisation techniques can help in the interpretation and validation of machine learning models, particularly when dealing with complex and non-linear models. The chapter also introduces a new method for dimensionality reduction in biomedical data analysis, called UMAP, and compares it with a more interpretable method, PCA. The results demonstrate the potential of using interactive visualisations to enhance understanding and trust in machine learning models, which could ultimately improve decision-making in the medical domain.

Finally, Chapter 10 continues the discussion on the broader aspect of visual communication and user trust in the health domain. In the health domain, building trust with users and patients is critical, as conservative attitudes and domain knowledge can outweigh the validity of analytical methods and processes. Visual communication and interaction are essential for enhancing trust and understanding, but trust issues still exist in current computational analytics and visualisation. This chapter explores the association of analytical processes with trust levels and provides guidance on improving interpretability and trust in health models and visualisations. By evaluating user expectations through interactive visualisation, the chapter aims to improve trust and understanding in the health domain.

0.3 CONCLUSION

The topic of data-driven science as applied to clinical healthcare is a broad and ever-expanding field for computational scientists. Yet how this will impact the health and biomedical domains, specifically at the clinical interface where such analytics impact daily medical decisions for patients, is not yet apparent, nor is it in active application within our medical centres. Whilst this book does not propose to be a comprehensive view of the entire field, we are pleased to present to you a series of chapters that demonstrate efforts to bring data-driven sciences into the healthcare domains so as to make a difference to our clinical practices and hence, eventually, improve the lives and wellbeing of patients.

Daniel R. Catchpoole
Simeon J. Simoff
Paul J. Kennedy
Quang Vinh Nguyen

Understanding the Impact of Patient Journey Patterns on Health Outcomes for Patients with Diabetes

Jamil Daher, Patricia Correll,
Paul J. Kennedy, and Barry Drake

1.1 INTRODUCTION

There is an increasing strain on health systems as a result of ageing populations as well as rising rates of obesity and other chronic disease risk factors [1]. In the United States, chronic conditions are responsible for seven out of ten deaths [2] and cost the economy over US$1 trillion annually [3]. This issue is not solely localised to the United States. For example, 47.3% of Australians suffer from at least one chronic condition [4]. Of particular concern has been diabetes, with around 11.1% of people in the state of New South Wales (NSW) estimated to have diabetes in 2018. These people experienced over 1.2 million episodes of care in the five-year period 2013–14 to 2018–19, with a significant number of these episodes relating to complications of diabetes [5]. As a result, there is a need to discover insights from patient journey data that can be used to enhance current treatment and management protocols.

NSW has a population of approximately 8.2 million and is Australia's largest state by population. Around 64.5% of residents are located within

DOI: 10.1201/9781003292357-1

the Greater Sydney region [6], where access to healthcare and socioeconomic advantage is greatest. As in other states, the NSW State Government is responsible for the delivery of acute care services, such as hospital inpatient, outpatient, and emergency services. While there exist privately run acute care services, most patients in NSW receive acute care in a public setting with 60% of hospitalisations occurring in public hospitals [7]. Primary care is typically provided by privately run GPs. There are 2840 GPs in NSW, of which over 500 provide data to Lumos.

Medicare is Australia's national health insurance scheme. Through the Medicare Benefits Scheme, most primary care services across Australia are provided to patients at either a heavily discounted price or for free. As a result, primary care services are readily accessible to most patients, with 88% of Australians attending a GP at least once in 2018–19 [8]. GPs in NSW are organised by location into one of ten primary health network (PHNs) regions. These are federally funded, independent organisations that are responsible for supporting and coordinating primary care services, as well as assessing the needs of the local population in their area, so that the delivery of care can be adjusted accordingly [9].

Researchers now have unprecedented access to many large datasets that have the potential to provide new insights into how people interact with the health system and associations with patient outcomes and experiences. An example of such a dataset is Lumos, which, at the time of this study, contained the records of over 2.8 million general practice (GP) patients in NSW linked to records in hospitals, emergency departments, and other medical services [10].

Past research has explored the impact of care at the GP on patient outcomes. Hernandez et al. [11] investigated whether follow-up hospital visits with a physician within seven days of an initial hospitalisation for heart failure reduced 30-day rehospitalisation rates. The results indicated a significant positive relationship between physician follow-ups and rehospitalisation rates. On the contrary, Zabawa et al. [12] and Hess et al. [13] both looked at the impact of GP visits on readmissions among patients with acute myocardial infarction in France and the United States, respectively. Neither found a significant relationship and concluded this may indicate differences in the effect of GP follow-up on acute versus chronic conditions. While studies have looked at the relationship between GP care and patient health outcomes for patients with various chronic conditions, very few studies have focused specifically on diabetes patients.

This chapter presents key findings from a retrospective cohort study of diabetes patients from general practices, examining associations between primary care events and patient outcomes. Several primary care events were studied, such as first antidiabetic prescription, health assessments, and general practice management plans. The patient outcomes considered were 28-day readmissions, unplanned hospital admissions, and mortality.

In the next section, we will describe the study methodology. We cover the patient cohort, data source, outcome measures, study factors, and analysis approach employed in our research. Following the methodology, we will present the key findings and discuss their implications. This chapter will conclude with a short summary.

1.2 METHODOLOGY

We used Lumos data to conduct a retrospective cohort analysis of people flagged with a diabetes diagnosis (in either a hospital or GP setting) between January 2011 and March 2020. We explored multiple study factors such as the delay in a patient acquiring their first antidiabetic prescription, GP visits immediately following an initial hospitalisation, and telehealth appointments. For each of these study factors, we looked for associations with three patient health outcomes: 28-day readmissions, unplanned hospital admissions, and mortality within five years of receiving a diabetes diagnosis.

1.2.1 Data Source

Our study analysed linked patient records from the Lumos dataset. The Lumos dataset was formed as part of a collaboration between NSW Ministry of Health and NSW Primary Health Networks (PHNs) to link the records of patients attending participating GPs to records in hospitals, emergency departments, and other medical services [10]. It contains records from patients who attended a participating GP at least once since January 2010 and includes data from patients across all 10 PHN regions in NSW. Data extraction and linkage are conducted twice per year in order to update the Lumos dataset with the latest available data. Lumos data is not publicly available and is only accessible via the Secure Analytics Primary Health Environment (SAPHE) provided by NSW Ministry of Health. As of March 2022, 561 GPs have enrolled in the Lumos program, encompassing 21% of all NSW GPs. These GPs provided the records of over 2.8 million patients that had attended their practice since January 2010. Past research has found Lumos data to be highly representative of the NSW population in terms of the distributions of age, sex, Index of Relative Socioeconomic Advantage and Disadvantage (IRSAD), and Accessibility and Remoteness Index of Australia (ARIA) [10].

1.2.2 Study Cohort

The study included all patients available in the Lumos dataset at the time of the study who had been diagnosed with diabetes between January 2011 and March 2020. The resultant cohort was 115,663 patients diagnosed with diabetes. Patients were classified as diabetic if they were flagged as having a diabetes diagnosis in their GP record or had been admitted to hospital and it was recorded that they had a principal or additional diagnosis of diabetes in their Admitted Patient (AP) record. While the diabetes diagnosis flags do not distinguish between the different types of diabetes, it is likely that most of these patients were diagnosed with type 2 diabetes, as other types of diabetes are relatively rare. Patients were only included in this study if they were flagged to have linked records in both the GP and AP datasets.

Table 1.1 describes each of the study factors included in our analysis. These study factors were chosen due to their relevance to the research questions and ease of interpretation. All events related to study factors, such as GP visits and prescription events, that occurred after a patient's diagnosis were extracted from the AP, GP, and Medication tables in the Lumos dataset. Telehealth GP appointments, as well as GP visits that involved either a health assessment or the development of a GP management plan, were identified by using the Medicare Benefits Schedule (MBS) billing codes associated with each GP event. The relevant MBS codes associated with these events have also been included in Table 1.1.

1.2.3 Timeframes

Each line of inquiry consisted of relevant study factor events (such as prescription events) and outcome events (such as unplanned hospital admissions) that occurred within a time period, described next. For most lines of inquiry, the date range for study factor events and outcome events was January 2011 to December 2019. Events from January 2020 onwards were excluded, as it is likely that the COVID-19 pandemic significantly impacted the GP usage patterns of patients. There were two exceptions to these rules.

First, for the first antidiabetic script delay, we looked at all outcome events between January 2011 and December 2019. However, we only

TABLE 1.1   Description of Study Factors Included in Analysis

Study Factor	Description
GP visit within seven days of hospitalisation	Flag for whether a patient visited a GP within seven days of discharge from an initial hospitalisation event (referred to as the index hospitalisation).
GP visit within 14 days of hospitalisation	Flag for whether a patient visited a GP within 14 days of discharge from an initial hospitalisation event (referred to as the index hospitalisation).
Mean GP visits per year (decile)	The average number of GP visits per year, grouped by decile, for a particular patient. A higher decile represents more frequent GP visits.
Index of dispersion for time between GP visits (decile)	The index of dispersion is defined as the ratio of variance to mean. In this scenario, it represents the normalised variation in the time between GP visits for each patient. The index of dispersion is grouped by decile, with a higher decile representing a larger index of dispersion and, consequently, less consistent visits to a GP.
Trend direction for time between GP visits	Represents whether the time between GP visits for a particular patient changed or stayed constant over time. Calculated using the gradient of a linear regression line fitted to the time between GP visits for each patient. A patient was considered to have a trend of increasing time between GP visits (indicating that GP visits became less frequent over time) if they had a gradient ≥ 1, a trend of decreasing time between GP visits if they had a gradient ≤ -1, and a constant trend otherwise.
First antidiabetic script delay	Amount of time between a patient's diagnosis and the date of first prescription for antidiabetic medication. First script delays were grouped into five categories: no script delay, 0–1 months script delay, 1–3 months script delay, 6–12 months script delay, and >1 year script delay.
GP management plan	Flag for whether a patient has had a GP management plan (MBS code 721) prepared for them. A GP management plan sets health goals agreed upon by both a patient and GP and describes the actions required to achieve these health goals.
Health assessment	Flag for whether a patient has received a health assessment (MBS codes 701, 703, 705, and 707). Health assessments involve examining a patient's condition and providing a preventive healthcare management plan for patients at risk of developing chronic conditions such as diabetes.
Past telehealth use	Flag for whether a patient has previously used telehealth GP services (MBS codes 91790, 91795, 91800-91802, and 91809-918011).

included prescription events that occurred between January 2011 and December 2018. The reason for this decision was to ensure that there was at least one year between a patient receiving their first antidiabetic prescription and the end of the study period. This allowed for evaluation of the relationship between script delay and unplanned admissions that occurred both before and after a patient was prescribed their first anti-diabetic medication. Secondly, data for telehealth events did not exist before March 2020. Therefore, when analysing the relationship between telehealth use and patient health outcomes, we looked at telehealth and outcome events that occurred between March 2020 and March 2021.

The time periods from which relevant study factor events and outcome events were extracted are detailed in Table 1.2.

The date ranges for diabetes diagnosis also varied by study factor and outcome measure. For most study factors, we included patients diagnosed between January 2011 and December 2017 when using unplanned hospital admissions as an outcome factor and January 2011 and December 2014 when using mortality within five years of diagnosis as an outcome factor. This guaranteed a time span of at least two and five years for each patient when looking at rates of unplanned admissions and mortality within five years of diagnosis, respectively, and allowed for more accurate calculation of the rates of outcome measures. There was one exception to this; as we only looked at telehealth events from March 2020 onwards, we included all patients diagnosed between January 2011 and March 2020 when looking at the impact of telehealth usage on patient health outcomes. Date ranges for diabetes diagnosis have also been included in Table 1.2.

1.2.4 Outcome Measures

Our study focused on the relationship between study factors and rates of unplanned hospital admissions and mortality within five years of receiving a diabetes diagnosis. Additionally, we looked at whether GP visits within 7 and 14 days of discharge from an initial hospitalisation were correlated with a decrease in 28-day readmission rates. A complete list of study factors for each outcome is included in Table 1.3.

1.2.5 Statistical Analysis

All relationships and trends uncovered were validated via statistical analysis at a 5% statistical significance level. When comparing the rates of outcomes across two categories, a two-sample Z-test was used to identify whether the observed results were statistically significant. When comparing the rates

TABLE 1.2   Date Ranges of Events and Diabetes Diagnosis for Each Study Factor

Study Factor	Date Ranges for Study Factor Events and Outcome Events	Date Ranges for Patient Diabetes Diagnosis
GP visit within seven days of hospitalisation	Jan 2011–Dec 2019	Jan 2011–Dec 2017
GP visit within 14 days of hospitalisation	Jan 2011–Dec 2019	Jan 2011–Dec 2017
Mean GP visits per year (decile)	Jan 2011–Dec 2019	Jan 2011–Dec 2017
Index of dispersion for time between GP visits (decile)	Jan 2011–Dec 2019	Jan 2011–Dec 2017
Trend direction for time between GP visits	Jan 2011–Dec 2019	Jan 2011–Dec 2017
First antidiabetic script delay	Jan 2011–Dec 2018 (for prescription events) Jan 2011–Dec 2019 (for outcome events)	Jan 2011–Dec 2017 (for unplanned admissions) Jan 2011–Dec 2014 (for mortality within five years of diagnosis)
GP management plan	Jan 2011–Dec 2019	Jan 2011–Dec 2017 (for unplanned admissions) Jan 2011–Dec 2014 (for mortality within five years of diagnosis)
Health assessment	Jan 2011–Dec 2019	Jan 2011–Dec 2017 (for unplanned admissions) Jan 2011–Dec 2014 (for mortality within five years of diagnosis)
Past telehealth use	Mar 2020–Mar 2021	Jan 2011–Mar 2020

TABLE 1.3   Study Factors Analysed for Each Patient Health Outcome

Outcome Measure	Study Factors
28-day readmission rate	GP visit within 7 days of hospitalisation GP visit within 14 days of hospitalisation
Mean yearly unplanned hospital admissions	Mean GP visits per year Index of dispersion for time between GP visits Trend direction for time between GP visits First antidiabetic script delay GP management plan Health assessment Past telehealth use
Mortality rate within 5 years of diagnosis	First antidiabetic script delay GP management plan Health assessment

of outcomes across three or more categories, conducting multiple Z-tests between each category will result in inflated Type I error rates. In order to combat this, a one-way ANOVA test was used to confirm that a difference in health outcomes existed initially. Post hoc analysis was performed using Tukey tests to identify where these differences exist precisely. Tukey tests were chosen specifically for their ability to calculate all pairwise differences without inflating the Type I error rate [14].

To confirm that observed relationships between study factors and patient health outcomes could not be explained by the presence of other confounding variables, multivariate logistic and linear regression models were built to compare the impact of variables to three demographic attributes: age, sex, and smoking status (reported as either 'Never Smoked', 'Ex-Smoker', 'Smoker', or 'Not Recorded'). Socio-economic status, as measured by the Socio-Economic Indexes for Areas (SEIFA), was included in our original analysis. However, SEIFA measures were later removed, as they did not provide any material benefit to the analysis. We produced plots of regression coefficients, with z-normalisation applied to all continuous variables to ensure that coefficients for variables were comparable. These plots provide a visual comparison of the impact of each variable on patient health outcomes.

1.3 RESULTS

1.3.1 28-Day Readmissions

Table 1.4 shows 28-day unplanned readmission rates according to whether a patient visited a GP within 7 or 14 days of initial hospitalisation. The results indicated higher 28-day readmission rates among patients who visited a GP after an initial hospitalisation. Compared to patients who did not visit a GP after a hospitalisation, patients who visited their GP within 7 and 14 days of discharge experienced approximately 43% and 28% more 28-day readmissions, respectively.

1.3.2 Unplanned Hospital Admissions

We found a moderately high frequency of GP visits correlated with lower rates of unplanned hospital admissions. Patients in deciles 5–8 (4.8–12.4 GP visits per year) experienced on average 27.5% fewer unplanned hospital admissions per year compared to patients in deciles 1–4 (0–4.8 GP visits per year) (Figure 1.1). Multivariate analysis further confirmed these results, with deciles 5–8 for GP visit frequency being the only significant features correlated with a reduction in rates of unplanned admissions

TABLE 1.4 28-Day Readmission Rates by Visits to GP within 7 or 14 Days of Discharge

Max Days Threshold for GP Visit	No GP Visit		GP Visit		Relative Risk	P-value
	28-Day Readmission Rate	Sample Size	28-Day Readmission Rate	Sample Size		
Seven Days	0.0647	537,060	0.0928	83,200	1.4343	<0.001
14 Days	0.0654	519,976	0.0843	100,284	1.2890	<0.001

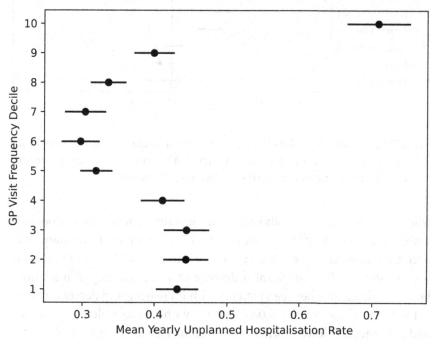

FIGURE 1.1   Mean and 95% CI for yearly unplanned hospital admission rate by GP visit frequency decile.

(Figure 1.2). However, rates of unplanned hospital admissions began to increase for patients with high to very high frequency of GP visits (beyond decile 8—over 12.4 GP visits per year), with patients in decile 10 (over 17 GP visits per year) experiencing 63.8% more unplanned hospital admissions per year than patients in deciles 1–4 (p-value < 0.001).

Patients who visited their GP more often or less often over time had slightly fewer unplanned hospitalisations per year compared to patients

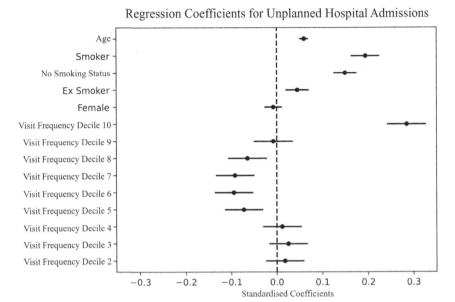

FIGURE 1.2 Coefficient plots (with 95% CI) from linear regression model containing GP visit frequency decile as a predictor. All continuous variables are normalised. Outcome measure is yearly unplanned admissions.

whose time between GP visits remained constant (relative risk of 'Constant' with 'Increasing' as reference category = 1.17, relative risk of 'Constant' with 'Decreasing' as reference category = 1.17, p-value < 0.001) (Figure 1.3). There was no statistically significant difference in the frequency of unplanned hospital admissions between patients with increasing and decreasing time between GP visits (p-value > 0.9). Patients with a lower index of dispersion and consequently lower normalised variability in the frequency of GP visits experienced higher rates of unplanned hospital admissions (Figure 1.4). Patients belonging to deciles 4–8 experienced between 21.6% and 63.4% less unplanned admissions per year compared to patients in deciles 1–3 (p-value < 0.001). The standardised coefficient plots produced by our multivariate analysis also showed lower rates of unplanned admissions among patients with a higher index of dispersion or a non-constant trend for the time between GP visits (Figures 1.5 and 1.6).

There was a considerable difference in unplanned admission rates between patients with no first script delay and patients who acquired their first script within one month of diagnosis. Patients who received their first script for an antidiabetic on the same day as their diagnosis experienced

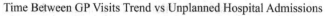

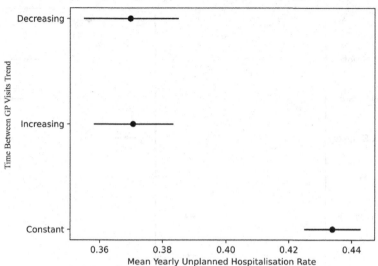

FIGURE 1.3 Mean and 95% CI for yearly unplanned hospital admission rate by trend of time between GP visits.

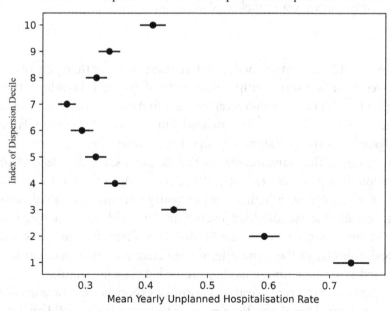

FIGURE 1.4 Mean and 95% CI for yearly unplanned hospital admission rate by index of dispersion decile.

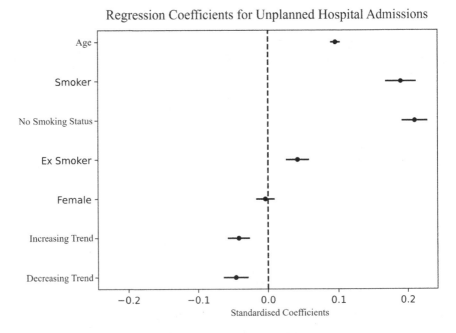

FIGURE 1.5 Coefficient plots (with 95% CI) from linear regression model containing GP visit trend as a predictor. All continuous variables are normalised. Outcome measure is yearly unplanned admissions.

on average 42% less unplanned hospitalisations per year than patients who received their first script within one month of diagnosis (p-value < 0.001) (Figure 1.7). All patients who received their first prescription for an antidiabetic after their diagnosis experienced similar rates of yearly unplanned admissions, with no statistically significant differences between any of these groups. The standardised coefficient plots showed a delayed prescription for a patient's first antidiabetic being one of the most important factors associated with higher rates of yearly unplanned hospitalisations (Figure 1.8). The standardised coefficient for a delayed first script was 2.8–3.5 times larger than the standardised coefficient for age and was statistically similar to the standardised coefficient for a patient either being reported as a smoker or not having a recorded smoking status.

Patients who received a health assessment experienced, on average, 24% more unplanned hospitalisations per year than patients who did not have a health assessment (Table 1.5). Our multivariate analysis also showed health assessments as a significant predictor of unplanned admission rates, with

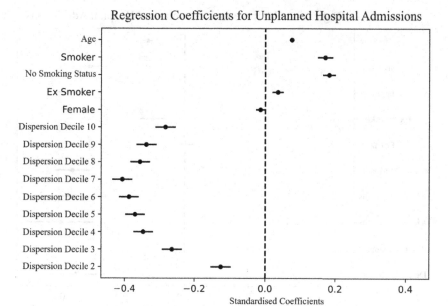

FIGURE 1.6   Coefficient plots (with 95% CI) from linear regression model containing index of dispersion as a predictor. All continuous variables are normalised. Outcome measure is yearly unplanned admissions.

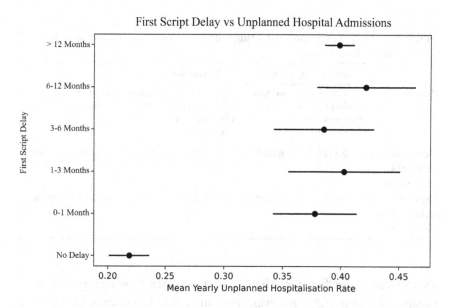

FIGURE 1.7   Mean and 95% CI for yearly unplanned hospital admission rate by first antidiabetic script delay.

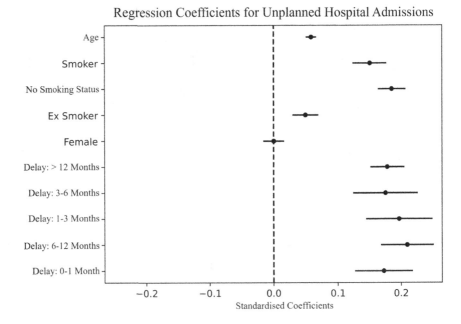

FIGURE 1.8 Coefficient plots (with 95% CI) from linear regression model containing first antidiabetic script delay as a predictor. All continuous variables are normalised. Outcome measure is yearly unplanned admissions.

TABLE 1.5 Mean Yearly Unplanned Hospital Admission Rates and Mortality Rates by Usage of Health Assessments

	No Health Assessment		Health Assessment			
Measure	Rate of Hospital Admissions or Mortality	Sample Size	Rate of Hospital Admissions or Mortality	Sample Size	Relative Risk	P-value
Mean yearly unplanned admissions	0.4117	64566	0.5128	9897	1.2456	**<0.001**
Mortality rates within five years	0.0475	41394	0.0687	6651	1.4463	**<0.001**

a standardised coefficient similar to age and a patient being reported as an ex-smoker (Figure 1.9). However, the standardised coefficient for a patient receiving a health assessment was approximately 70% less than the standardised coefficient for a patient being reported as a smoker, suggesting

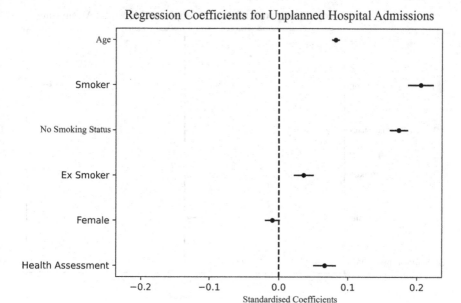

FIGURE 1.9 Coefficient plots (with 95% CI) from linear regression model containing the health assessment flag as a predictor. All continuous variables are normalised. Outcome measure is yearly unplanned admissions.

TABLE 1.6 Mean Yearly Unplanned Hospital Admission Rates and Mortality Rates by Usage of GP Management Plans

| Measure | No GP Management Plan | | GP Management Plan | | | |
	Rate of Hospital Admissions or Mortality	Sample Size	Rate of Hospital Admissions or Mortality	Sample Size	Relative Risk	P-value
Mean yearly unplanned admissions	0.4742	42196	0.3610	32267	0.7613	**<0.001**
Mortality rates within five years	0.0652	26682	0.0320	21363	0.4908	**<0.001**

that receiving a health assessment was a relatively insignificant predictor of yearly unplanned admissions in comparison to a patient's smoking status.

On the other hand, patients who received GP management plans experienced, on average, 24% fewer unplanned admissions per year compared to patients who did not have a GP management plan (Table 1.6). The

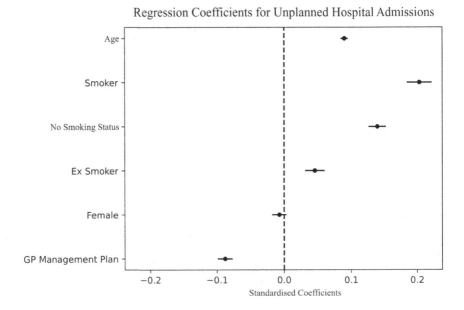

FIGURE 1.10   Coefficient plots (with 95% CI) from linear regression model containing the GP management plan flag as a predictor. All continuous variables are normalised. Outcome measure is yearly unplanned admissions.

standardised coefficient plot in Figure 1.10 provides further validation to this result, showing that GP management plans significantly correlated with decreased rates of unplanned admissions. Comparing absolute standardised coefficients, GP management plans had a comparable impact to age on rates of unplanned admissions.

The use of telehealth was correlated with 17.6% higher rates of unplanned hospital admission (p-value < 0.001) (Table 1.7). Further analysis by plotting the standardised coefficients reveals that telehealth usage had similar levels of impact on unplanned hospitalisation rates to ex-smoking status and age (Figure 1.11). However, a patient being reported as a smoker had a three times higher impact on predicted unplanned hospitalisation rates compared to telehealth usage, suggesting that smoking is an important modifier in these analyses.

1.3.3 Mortality

A delayed first prescription for an antidiabetic was correlated with higher rates of mortality within five years of diagnosis. Patients who acquired

TABLE 1.7   Mean Yearly Unplanned Hospital Admission Rate by Telehealth Usage

Measure	No Telehealth Usage		Used Telehealth		Relative Risk	P-value
	Rate of Hospital Admissions or Mortality	Sample Size	Rate of Hospital Admissions or Mortality	Sample Size		
Mean yearly unplanned admissions	0.2338	59383	0.2749	28488	1.1758	<0.001

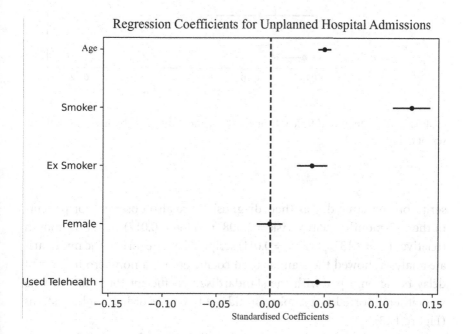

FIGURE 1.11   Coefficient plots (with 95% CI) from linear regression model containing the telehealth flag as a predictor. All continuous variables are normalised. Outcome measure is yearly unplanned hospital admissions.

their first script at least a year after diagnosis were approximately 2.5 times more likely to die within five years of diagnosis than patients who acquired their first script on the same day as their diabetes diagnosis (p-value < 0.001) (Figure 1.12). At a 5% significance level, statistically significant differences in rates of mortality compared to patients who acquired their first

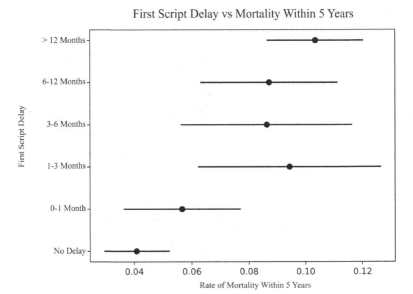

FIGURE 1.12   Mean and 95% CI for five-year mortality rate by first antidiabetic script delay.

script on the same day as their diagnosis were also observed for patients in the 1–3-month (relative risk = 2.308, p-value = 0.017) and 6–12-month (relative risk = 2.132, p-value = 0.011) script delay categories. The multivariate analysis showed the standardised coefficient for a non-zero first script delay being on a par with the standardised coefficient for a patient who was either reported as a smoker or did not have a recorded smoking status (Figure 1.13).

We observed 44% higher rates of mortality within five years of diagnosis among patients who received a health assessment (Table 1.5). However, the standardised coefficient plots indicated that health assessments were correlated with a significant decrease in mortality rates (odds ratio = 0.613), with age responsible for much of the increase in rates of mortality (Figure 1.14). Further analysis revealed that patients who received a health assessment were approximately 14 years older on average and therefore more at risk of dying. Patients who had a prepared GP management plan experienced 51% lower rates of mortality within five years of diagnosis (Table 1.6), with the standardised coefficients produced from the multivariate analysis further supporting these findings (Figure 1.15).

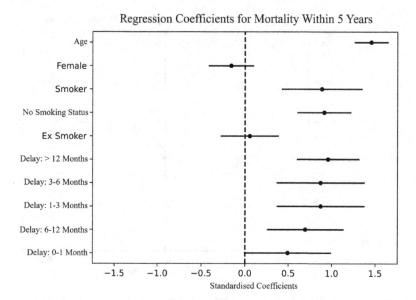

FIGURE 1.13   Coefficient plots (with 95% CI) from logistic regression model containing first antidiabetic script delay as a predictor. All continuous variables are normalised. Outcome measure is mortality within five years of diagnosis.

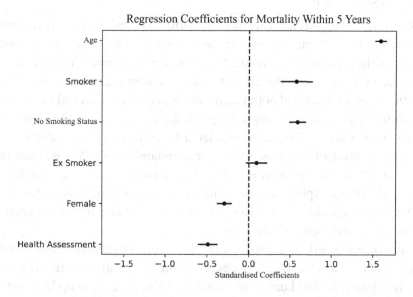

FIGURE 1.14   Coefficient plots (with 95% CI) from logistic regression model containing the health assessment flag as a predictor. All continuous variables are normalised. Outcome measure is mortality within five years of diagnosis.

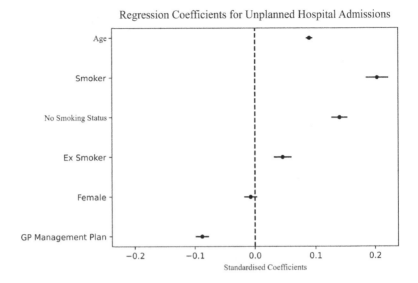

FIGURE 1.15   Coefficient plots (with 95% CI) from logistic regression model containing the GP management plan flag as a predictor. All continuous variables are normalised. Outcome measure is mortality within five years of diagnosis.

1.4 DISCUSSION

Our study highlights key contributors within a primary care setting that affect health outcomes for patients with diabetes. We found shorter first script delays, moderately frequent GP visits, more variation in the time between GP visits, and the use of GP management plans were associated with decreases in rates of both yearly unplanned admissions and mortality within five years of receiving a diagnosis for diabetes. GP visits immediately after a hospitalisation were related to an increase in 28-day readmission rates. Health assessments were correlated with increased rates of both unplanned admissions and mortality. However, multivariate analysis showed that age explained most of the increase in mortality rates. Patients who used telehealth GP services at least once were also found to experience more unplanned admissions.

A major strength of our study was the use of a large, population-based linked dataset to ascertain activities across the care continuum that impact patient journeys. The Lumos data asset provides a regularly updated data resource that can deliver unique insights about statewide, cross-setting healthcare utilisation. General practice patients included in the Lumos data asset have been shown to be representative of the NSW population [10]. The work presented here was limited to the subset of patients with diabetes who had experienced at least one hospital admission in Lumos data. Further work is required to explore the impact of this restriction and the relationship between primary care events and health outcomes for patients with diabetes who did not have any recorded hospital admissions.

Our study supports earlier prescription of antidiabetic medication in order to ensure better health outcomes for patients with diabetes. To the best of our knowledge, this is the first study to analyse the relationship between first antidiabetic script delays and patient health outcomes. Longer first script delays may be a sign of patients who forgo medication in favour of diet and exercise to manage their diabetic condition, as well as patients who are simply less proactive in acquiring treatment. While a prescription alone does not necessarily indicate adherence to a medication plan, it may be easier to adhere to a medication plan than it is to adhere to a rigorous diet and exercise plan. As a result, it is expected that patients with a shorter script delay experience better health outcomes.

Interestingly, however, a substantial difference in unplanned admission rates existed between patients who acquired their first script on the same day as their diagnosis and patients who acquired their first script within one month of diagnosis. Additionally, all patients who received their first script after their diagnosis date experienced similar rates of unplanned admissions. The reason for these results is unclear. Nonetheless, our findings indicate that patients with diabetes who acquired their first antidiabetic script earlier experienced better health outcomes with respect to unplanned hospital admissions and mortality.

Patterns of engagement with GPs were also significantly associated with patient health outcomes. Patients who visited GPs with moderate to high frequency were shown to experience fewer unplanned admissions. This is unsurprising, as GP visits allow for a patient to regularly monitor their condition and treat underlying issues before they require hospitalisation. Previous research using Lumos data found lower rates of unplanned admissions among patients who visited GPs that had a higher overall frequency of visits from patients [15]. Our study is consistent with these findings using patient-level visitation rates instead of practice-level visitation rates. The observation that patients who visited GPs with very high frequency (17+ times per year) also had more unplanned admissions is likely to reflect patients at the extreme end of the disease spectrum, with advanced or complex health needs resulting in higher demand across the healthcare continuum.

Our findings support the idea that patients who do not require regular GP visits often experience better health outcomes. Patients who visited their GP less consistently, as measured through the index of dispersion for the time between GP visits, experienced fewer unplanned admissions. One explanation for this finding is that patients who do not require consistent GP visits have less severe health impairment. Consequently, these patients experience fewer unplanned admissions. Patients who visited their GP either more frequently or less frequently after their diagnosis also experienced lower rates of unplanned admissions than people who visited their GP at a constant rate. This may be for a similar reason as why there were fewer unplanned admissions amongst patients with a higher index of dispersion for the time between GP visits. Patients with a non-constant GP visit trend can also be viewed as patients who are less consistent with how often they visit their GP due to better management of their condition. By extension, these patients should experience fewer negative health events. As this measure only captures the linear trend in the time between GP visits, it is unable to capture more subtle trends, such as whether a patient visited their GP more frequently for a short period of time before returning to normal levels of GP visit frequency. Even with our blunt approach, we were able to discover valuable insights. Future analysis might refine this approach further to explore the relationship between GP visit trends and health outcomes in more detail.

We found GP visits within 7 and 14 days of an initial hospitalisation associated with increased rates of 28-day readmissions. This contrasts with other analyses in Lumos data addressing similar questions that produced findings in the opposite direction [16]. The other analyses were not specific to diabetes, so the difference may be a feature of the patient journeys of people with diabetes. However, the difference may relate to methodology. In our methodological approach, we did not exclude cases where readmission occurred within 7 or 14 days of discharge from an initial hospitalisation, whereas the other Lumos analyses excluded these readmissions to separate the time periods for ascertaining the exposure and outcome. Further work is needed to understand the differences in these results.

Elsewhere, research looking at the impact of GP visits on readmission rates has also generated mixed findings. Patients hospitalised for chronic heart failure were found to be less likely to be readmitted if they had follow-up physician visits at a hospital [11]. On the other hand, no significant reduction in readmission rates was observed for patients with acute myocardial infarctions (AMIs) who visited a GP or hospital physician after an initial hospitalisation event [2, 13]. One reason suggested for the lack of change in readmission rates for AMI patients was that GP visits are not able to prevent deterioration in the short term for acute conditions such as AMI. While diabetes is a chronic rather than acute condition, a similar line of reasoning could be applied in that GP visits are more effective as a tool for long-term rather than short-term improvement in a patient's condition. Another reason for the increase in readmission rates amongst patients with diabetes who visited a GP after an initial hospitalisation may be that a GP visit allowed for the identification of unmet needs that required medical attention in an acute setting.

Having a GP management plan prepared was a strong indicator of both lower unplanned admission rates and lower rates of mortality within five years of diagnosis. GP management plans are a more direct method of managing a patient's diabetic condition, as through the preparation of a plan, clear management goals are set, and arrangements are made for providing the necessary services required to achieve the management goals. Therefore, it is not surprising to see that GP management plans positively impact patient health outcomes.

The univariate and multivariate analyses indicate that health assessments were correlated with a slight increase in unplanned admission rates. Health assessments are recommended for patients with risk factors that increase their likelihood of developing a chronic condition. It is plausible that the increase in unplanned admissions is simply a consequence of unmet needs being identified and appropriately addressed. Our study included a limited number of attributes in our multivariate analysis. As such, it is possible that other variables, such as a patient having comorbidities, may explain the increase in unplanned hospital admissions for patients who received a health assessment. Our univariate analysis also highlighted an increase in mortality rates for patients who received a health assessment. However, our multivariate analysis revealed that much of this increase in mortality rates was attributable to age, as these patients were 14 years older on average.

Our study found telehealth usage related to a slight increase in unplanned admission rates. GP telehealth items first became available in March 2020. As a result, unplanned admission rates were calculated for this analysis using only one year of data. Future analysis with a larger span of data may yield a different result. Two other limitations arose as a result of the short duration of telehealth data.

- We were unable to study the impact of the frequency of telehealth usage on patient health outcomes. Our study found that unplanned hospital admission rates varied significantly according to the level of engagement with GP services. It is possible that the frequency of telehealth usage follows a similar trend.

- The relationship between telehealth usage and mortality rates could not be evaluated.

1.5 CONCLUSION

The structure of the Australian health system complicates the flow of data across the healthcare continuum because it is collected by different arms of government as well as by private organisations. Therefore, 'whole of system' data is not available in one place, while from the patient perspective, activities and outcomes of one part of the health sector are often most apparent in another. This is especially the case in general practice where GP activities occur between episodes of other types of healthcare.

The Lumos program addresses this by providing unique linked data across the healthcare continuum that transcends the differing governmental and private structures. This data can be used to reveal important insights about patient healthcare journeys. Here we have demonstrated this in the context of diabetes care in NSW, focusing on activities in general practice and outcomes in acute care and mortality. Our study identified many aspects of a diabetic patient's engagement with GP services associated with either an improvement or worsening of health outcomes. Future study could further explore age specific death rates factored by different age groups.

By highlighting the ways in which a patient's engagement with GP services influences health outcomes, these insights provide guidance to GPs and governments on how the delivery of healthcare can be improved. Additionally, our study paints a picture of how high-risk patients engage with GP services. This allows for targeted care to be provided to these individuals in order to positively alter the trajectory of their patient journey and future health outcomes. Finally, our study further validates the usefulness of linked patient records for generating clinically actionable knowledge.

ACKNOWLEDGEMENTS

The Lumos program is a partnership of the NSW Ministry of Health and NSW Primary Health Networks and is possible through the participation of general practices across NSW. Record linkage was carried out by the Centre for Health Record Linkage.

REFERENCES

1. U.S. Department of Health and Human Services. (2010). *Multiple Chronic Conditions—A Strategic Framework: Optimum Health and Quality of Life for Individuals with Multiple Chronic Conditions.* Washington: U.S. Department of Health and Human Services.
2. Partnership to Fight Chronic Diseases. (2007). *The Growing Crisis of Chronic Disease in the United States.* Retrieved April 9, 2022, from www.healthcatalyst.com/wp-content/uploads/2014/04/How-to-Improve-Patient-Outcomes.pdf
3. National Association of Chronic Disease Directors. (2012). *Why Public Health Is Necessary to Improve Healthcare.* Retrieved April 9, 2022, from https://chronicdisease.org/resource/resmgr/white_papers/cd_white_paper_hoffman.pdf
4. Australian Bureau of Statistics. (2018). *Chronic Conditions, 2017–18 Financial Year.* Retrieved April 9, 2022, from www.abs.gov.au/statistics/health/health-conditions-and-risks/chronic-conditions/2017–18
5. NSW Health. (2020). *Diabetes Management in NSW—Case for Change Summary.* Retrieved April 9, 2022, from www.health.nsw.gov.au/Value/Documents/diabetes-management-case-for-change-summary.pdf
6. NSW Government. (2020). *Key facts about NSW.* Retrieved April 9, 2022, from www.nsw.gov.au/about-nsw/key-facts-about-nsw
7. Australian Institute of Health and Welfare (2020). *Australia's Hospitals at a Glance: 2018–19.* Retrieved April 9, 2022 from www.aihw.gov.au/getmedia/c14c8e7f-70a3-4b00-918c-1f56d0bd9414/aihw-hse-247.pdf.aspx?inline=true
8. Australian Institute of Health and Welfare (2020). *Medicare-subsidised GP, Allied Health and Specialist Health Care across Local Areas: 2013–14 to 2018–19.* Retrieved April 9, 2022 from www.aihw.gov.au/reports/primary-health-care/medicare-subsidised-health-local-areas-2019/contents/gp-attendances/gp-attendances
9. Australian Government Department of Health. (2021). *What Primary Health Networks Are.* Retrieved April 9, 2022, from www.health.gov.au/initiatives-and-programs/phn/what-phns-are
10. Correll, P., Feyer, A.-M., Phan, P.-T., et al. (2021). Lumos: A statewide linkage programme in Australia integrating general practice data to guide system redesign. *Integrated Healthcare Journal, 3*(1)
11. Hernandez, A. (2010). Relationship between early physician follow-up and 30-day readmission among medicare beneficiaries hospitalized for heart failure. *JAMA, 303*(17), 1716–1722.
12. Zabawa, C., Cottenet, J., Zeller, M., Mercier, G., Rodwin, V., Cottin, Y., and Quantin, C. (2018). Thirty-day rehospitalizations among elderly patients with acute myocardial infarction. *Medicine, 97*(24), e11085.
13. Hess, C., Shah, B., Peng, S., Thomas, L., Roe, M., and Peterson, E. (2013). Association of early physician follow-up and 30-day readmission after non-ST-segment-elevation myocardial infarction among older patients. *Circulation, 128*(11), 1206–1213.

14. McHugh, M. L. (2011). Multiple comparison analysis testing in ANOVA. *Biochemia Medica*, 21(3), 203–209.
15. NSW Health. (2021). *General Practice Affecting Hospital Visits*. Retrieved April 9, 2022, from www.health.nsw.gov.au/lumos/Documents/gp-atten dance-affects-hospital-visits.pdf
16. NSW Health. (2022). *Lumos Factsheet: Care in General Practice Can Affect Hospital Visits*. Retrieved April 9, 2022, from www.health.nsw.gov.au/lumos/Factsheets/readmissions-to-hospital.pdf

CHAPTER 2

COVID-19 Impact Analysis on Patients with Complex Health Conditions

A Literature Review

Xueping Peng, Guodong Long, Peng Yan,
Wensi Tang, and Allison Clarke

2.1 INTRODUCTION

COVID-19 was first reported in December 2019 [1], and the World Health Organization (WHO) announced the pandemic in 2020 [2]. COVID-19 is very easily spread from person to person, similar to influenza. However, it is more deadly than the influenza. In 2020, there were a total of 82,661,679 people infected with COVID-19 and 1,879,763 deaths [3]. The impact of the pandemic gradually decreased in 2021 due to increasing vaccination coverage. To date, several countries have already opened their economies and borders with nearly full vaccination rates, and most of the others have published clear plans to relieve restrictions upon reaching vaccination coverage targets.

Governments in different countries have used a range of strategies to tackle the pandemic. Moreover, in different stages of the pandemic, the national response strategies changed according to real-world impacts. Most of these strategies restricted people's movements in the physical world. This type of restriction strategy caused substantial economic

DOI: 10.1201/9781003292357-2

losses to both the domestic and international economies. According to the International Labour Organization, in 2020, 8.8 per cent of global working hours were lost relative to the fourth quarter of 2019, which was equivalent to 255 million full-time jobs [4].

COVID-19 infections usually impact patients' upper respiratory systems, which makes them deadly. Even if patients recover from COVID-19, they can suffer some permanent side effects, such as fatigue and shortness of breath. Patients' families can experience mental health issues or illnesses due to the loss of family members or the need for ongoing care. Moreover, many people have also suffered from mental health issues caused by the pandemic, such as financial pressures, loss of work, restricted household visits and lack of face-to-face communication. In addition to these impacts, patients with complex health conditions are among the most vulnerable populations in the pandemic. People with compromised immune systems or pre-existing medical conditions, including cancer, may be at increased risk of contracting COVID-19 and more severe infections. Due to the impact of the COVID-19 pandemic, these people have reduced and delayed visits to clinicians and pathology testing. Therefore, healthcare for people with cancer may have been disrupted due to government policy decisions and limited health resources available during the COVID-19 pandemic.

Three kinds of patient groups are studied. The first group is patients with chronic diseases, such as diabetes, cardiovascular disease and severe mental illness. The second group is cancer patients who need continuous medical treatment to control the progression of the disease. The third group is patients receiving end-of-life care whose survival rate and quality of life are related to the quality of care received.

The pandemic's impact is studied using both qualitative and quantitative analytics. Medical-based quantitative analysis can give insights into the impact with logical reasoning, and data-driven qualitative analytics can provide evidence to support real-world impacts. With widespread digitisation and data collection techniques, many available datasets can be integrated to examine the impact on human life and services received. Moreover, the COVID-19 pandemic is also examined using various analytical methods, and these results and data sources may also be valuable for conducting impact analysis. Our main contributions are summarised as follows:

- This chapter surveys analytical work conducted on how COVID-19 has impacted patients with complex health conditions.

- We categorise vulnerable populations into three specific cohorts: patients with chronic disease, patients with cancer and patients with end-of-life care.

- We investigate how each of these cohorts has been impacted by the pandemic and identify each cohort from an analytics perspective by leveraging various data collection strategies and analytical methods.

The remainder of this chapter is organised as follows. Section 2.2 reviews related works. Then, three specific cohorts are categorised in Sections 2.3, 2.4 and 2.5. And next, in Section 2.6, we demonstrate the various data collection strategies and analytical methods. Last, we conclude the work in Section 2.7.

2.2 RELATED WORK

2.2.1 COVID-19–Related Analytics by the Australian Government

Key COVID-19 analytical publications include the Australian Institute of Health and Welfare's (AIHW) report on the impact of the COVID-19 pandemic on health and welfare issues relevant in Australia [5]. The Australian Government Department of Health has collected rich information to record statistical information on COVID-19–related activities [6]. The Treasury has also published a report on the impacts of COVID-19 [7].

The Australian Bureau of Statistics (ABS) has released a range of new statistical and research products to help understand the impacts of COVID-19 [8]. This includes additional analysis and information on economic statistics, including the classification of COVID-19 policies and selected issues in the economic accounts and method changes. Expanded integrated data resources have also been developed to inform the COVID-19 response through the Multi-Agency Data Integration Project (MADIP) [9].

For specific cohorts, some health organisations have conducted analysis on service providers in Australia in response to the COVID-19 pandemic. For example, Cancer Australia investigated Medicare Benefits Schedule (MBS) claims to understand the impact of COVID-19 on medical services and procedures in Australia [10]. Services for a range of diagnostic and therapeutic procedures were examined for the five highest incidences of cancers, breast, colorectal, lung, prostate and skin cancer-related services. The report showed substantial reductions in procedures relating to cancer investigations and treatments have been reported by service providers in Australia due to the COVID-19 pandemic.

2.2.2 Stringency Index

Governments have examined a wide range of measures in response to the COVID-19 pandemic. These tools have aimed to track and compare policy responses around the world rigorously and consistently. The Stringency Index [11] is one of the tools used to measure the governments' response metrics to COVID-19. This index was produced by the Oxford COVID-19 Government Response Tracker (OxCGRT) [12]. The index records the strictness of lockdown-style policies that primarily restrict people's behaviour. It is calculated using all ordinal containment and closure policy indicators as well as an indicator recording public information campaigns.

Australia has used the index to measure the government's response to COVID-19, and it stood at a 68.06 on 21 July 2021, according to Spectator Australia [13]. The ABS has applied the Stringency Index to each of Australia's eight states and territories, using archived official sources to rank the severity of restrictions on movement and the government's response. Eight indices have been produced to measure the stringency of a state/territory governments' responses to COVID-19, with a score of 100 indicating the maximum level of restrictions [14].

2.3 IMPACT ON PATIENTS WITH CHRONIC DISEASES

People with chronic conditions are at greater risk of more serious illnesses if they are infected with COVID-19. These people need protection from COVID-19 and should avoid exposure to the public if they are infected with the virus, which may disrupt their healthcare, such as scheduled appointments with their doctors. To facilitate the impact analysis of COVID-19, chronic diseases can be categorised as follows:

- High-incidence chronic conditions: cardiovascular disease, diabetes, kidney disease and respiratory disease

- Neurological conditions: epilepsy and multiple sclerosis

- Eye and macular diseases, such as anti–vascular endothelial growth factor (VEGF) treatment

- Musculoskeletal diseases

- Chronic pain

- Endometriosis

- HIV

- Hepatitis

- Osteoporosis

- Rare diseases, such as spinal muscular atrophy (SMA) and cystic fibrosis

- Severe mental illnesses, including schizophrenia, psychotic disorders, bipolar disorder and major depression.

2.3.1 Literature Review

High-incidence chronic conditions. Chronic conditions are an ongoing cause of substantial ill health, disability, and premature death, making them an important global, national and individual health concern. Also referred to as chronic diseases, non-communicable diseases or long-term health conditions, chronic conditions are generally characterised by long-lasting and persistent effects [15]. In this review, high-incidence chronic conditions include cardiovascular disease, diabetes, kidney and respiratory disease, and so on.

Cardiovascular diseases. COVID-19 patients with cardiovascular comorbidities are at higher risk of morbidity and mortality [16]. Myocardial injury (MI) is present in more than 25 per cent of critical cases and presents in two patterns: acute MI and dysfunction on presentation and MI that develops as the illness severity intensifies. Additionally, it has been shown that COVID-19 is associated with several cardiovascular complications, including MI and myocarditis, acute MI, heart failure, arrhythmia, stress-induced cardiomyopathy, venous thromboembolism (VTE), acute coronary syndrome and disseminated intravascular coagulation (DIC). There are concerns regarding how medications used to treat COVID-19 patients may lead to cardiovascular complications, and their use should be carefully considered before treating such patients [17]. Ref. [18] investigated the impact on the care of cardiovascular patients and the changes to hospital logistics that conflict with important principles for the treatment of acute coronary syndrome patients.

Diabetes. Diabetes has been reported as a determinant of severity and mortality for patients with COVID-19 [19]. To this end, a set of measures has been studied for patients with diabetes. For example, in Ref. [20], the authors compared phenotypic characteristics between in- and outpatients with diabetes mellitus and COVID-19 infections and established an easy-to-use hospitalisation prediction risk score. Ref. [21] studied potential mechanisms that increase the risk of COVID-19 in people with diabetes. Ref. [22] proposed a set of measures for patients of diabetes with COVID-19 infections, including specific and general preventive measures. They included, for example, hospitalised patients with severe disease needing frequent blood glucose monitoring.

Kidney disease. Clinical reports have shown that there is a remarkable fraction of patients admitted to hospitals due to COVID-19 with signs of kidney dysfunctions [23], including 59 per cent with proteinuria; 44 per cent with haematuria; 14 per cent with increased levels of blood urea nitrogen; and 10 per cent with increased levels of serum creatinine, mild but worse than that in cases with other pneumonia. A univariate Cox regression analysis showed that proteinuria, haematuria and elevated levels of blood urea nitrogen, serum creatinine and uric acid as well as D-dimer (a protein fragment that occurs when a blood clot dissolves in a person's body) were significantly associated with the death of COVID-19 patients. Importantly, the Cox regression analysis also suggested that COVID-19 patients who developed acute kidney injury (AKI) had 5.3 times the mortality risk of those without AKI, which is much higher than that of other comorbid chronic illnesses. AKI has been reported in up to 25 per cent of critically ill patients with COVID-19 infections, especially in those with underlying comorbidities [24].

Respiratory disease. Distinguishing between symptoms of COVID-19 and those resulting from other respiratory diseases is helpful when managing patients in hospital. Ref. [25] compared patients with and without COVID-19 who tested positive for another respiratory virus. They concluded that patients with COVID-19 reported longer symptom durations and were more often hospitalised, but most comorbidities, medications, symptoms, vital signs, laboratory test results, treatments and outcomes did not differ according to COVID-19 status. However, it is worth noting that the in-hospital mortality of patients with COVID-19 presenting with mild symptoms is higher and associated with older age, platelet count and ferritin levels. Identifying early predictors of the outcomes can be useful in clinical practices to better stratify and manage patients with COVID-19. Refs. [26] and [27] provided a compact overview of recommendations by the European Forum for Research and Education in Allergy and Airway Diseases (EUFOREA) expert teams on allergic airway diseases and allergen-specific immunotherapy (AIT). It deals with similarities and differences between allergic rhinitis (AR) and coronavirus infection and specific recommendations for allergic disease care in the COVID-19 era, including guidance on AIT. Ref. [28] investigated extra-respiratory manifestations to help clinicians better understand the range of clinical presentations associated with COVID-19.

Neurological conditions.

Epilepsy. Epilepsy is a disorder in which nerve cell activity in the brain is disturbed, causing seizures [29]. A medical history of epilepsy has not been reported as a risk factor for developing COVID-19. Moreover, past experiences with infectious diseases do not suggest any associations [30]. Ref. [31] summarised the current evidence on various effects of COVID-19 on epilepsy. Ref. [32] compared the severity of psychological distress between patients with epilepsy and healthy controls during the COVID-19 pandemic in southwest China and identified potential risk factors of severe psychological distress among patients with epilepsy. Ref. [33] provided a survey on epilepsy during COVID-19. They found that the COVID-19 pandemic has affected epilepsy patients. Patients with tumour-related, drug-resistant epilepsy; insomnia; and economic difficulties are at a higher risk of increased seizure frequency.

Multiple sclerosis. Multiple sclerosis (MS) is an autoimmune disease of the central nervous system. It interferes with nerve impulses within the brain, spinal cord and optic nerves [34]. Ref. [35] assessed the severity of COVID-19 in patients suffering from MS, Parkinson's disease and cognitive impairment through a questionnaire-based study. They found that none of the patients with COVID-19 confirmed by reverse transcription polymerase chain reaction (RT-PCR) developed clinical manifestations of infectious diseases. They also did not report any significant changes in neurological status during the course of the primary nervous system disease. Ref. [36] highlighted the implications of COVID-19 for people with MS and related disorders, including the risk of respiratory infections, general health advice and recommendations (from consensus-based guidelines) for immunotherapy, relapse management and service delivery during the COVID-19 pandemic. Ref. [37] recommended setting up a program to collect information to evaluate the relationship between MS and COVID-19 and implement immediate and appropriate protective strategies.

Eye and macular diseases. Eye disease causes vision loss. Macular degeneration causes loss in the centre of the field of vision. In dry macular degeneration, the centre of the retina deteriorates [38]. With wet macular degeneration, leaky blood vessels grow under the retina. Ref. [39] assessed the impact of the COVID-19 lockdown on the visual acuity and macular thickness of patients with macular oedema receiving intravitreal injections. Specifically, delayed intravitreal injections resulted in variable outcomes. Triaging the urgency of patients should be based on the equity principle of bioethics in which those in need are prioritised over others, depending on potential adverse outcomes. Ref. [40] provided a proof-of-concept calculation to determine the health-adjusted life-year trade-off between intravitreal anti-VEGF injections and the transmission of COVID-19. Clinical ophthalmological guidelines have encouraged the assessment of potential benefits and harms when deciding whether to perform elective ophthalmology procedures during the COVID-19 pandemic in order to minimise the risk of disease transmission.

Musculoskeletal diseases. Ref. [41] investigated temporal trends in COVID-19 outcomes in patients with rheumatic and musculoskeletal diseases over the course of the pandemic. The outcomes were assessed within 30 days of COVID-19 diagnosis, including hospitalisation, intensive care unit (ICU) admission, invasive mechanical ventilation, renal failure and death. To study the musculoskeletal consequences of COVID-19, Ref. [42] summarised the known musculoskeletal pathologies in patients with severe acute respiratory syndrome (SARS) or COVID-19 and combined them with computational modelling and biochemical signalling studies to predict musculoskeletal cellular targets and long-term consequences of the COVID-19. To provide guidance to rheumatology healthcare providers on the use of COVID-19 vaccines for patients with rheumatic and musculoskeletal diseases (RMD), Ref. [43] provided advice on the best use of COVID-19 vaccines and the implementation of vaccination strategies for RMD patients.

Chronic pain. Chronic pain is often part of the quality of life, but how this additional comorbidity affects critical care survivors is poorly understood. Estimates of chronic pain prevalence after ICU treatment vary from 14 to 77 per cent, depending on the time scale, method of measurement and population [44]. It is likely that those who survive critical illness from COVID-19 will be at particular risk of developing chronic pain Chronic pain must be considered in the context of a biopsychosocial model, which views symptoms resulting from complex and dynamic interactions between biological, psychological and social factors [45]. There are four related factors to help guide healthcare professionals caring for patients with chronic pain:

- the public health consequences of COVID-19 for patients with pain,

- the consequences of not treating these patients for the duration of this pandemic,

- options for remote assessment and management and

- clinical evidence supporting remote therapies [46,47].

Endometriosis. Endometriosis is a chronic pain condition in premenopausal women. A web-based cross-sectional survey [48] on the pain experience and social support of endometriosis patients during the COVID-19 pandemic was conducted in Germany. The survey findings showed that physical pain and disability on the one hand and emotional and social pain experienced on the other were affected differently by emotional, social and healthcare constraints related to the COVID-19 pandemic. The COVID-19 pandemic has led to a severe disruption in the clinical practice of women's health and routine care for endometriosis. Ref. [49] presented clinical advice on the management of endometriosis during the COVID-19 pandemic and future considerations.

HIV. The COVID-19 pandemic has presented several barriers and challenges to the HIV care continuum rather than the pressure it brings to people living with HIV [50]. Although there was a trend towards increased rates of ICU admission, mechanical ventilation and mortality in HIV-positive patients, these differences were not statistically significant [51]. However, COVID-19 has put significant pressure on the HIV care continuum. First, the implementation of quarantine, social distancing and community containment measures have reduced access to routine HIV testing. Testing remains a challenge in settings with scarce access to these kits. Therefore, increased efforts are needed to augment access and facilitate testing. Second, timely access to HIV care may have been hindered during the COVID-19 pandemic, as initiated antiretroviral therapy can be deterred or delayed because hospitals are busy treating patients with COVID-19. Due to global tension in the public health system, the allocation of resources for HIV care may have been diminished. Third, the COVID-19 pandemic may also have hindered antiretroviral therapy continuation.

Hepatitis. The World Hepatitis Alliance, a global umbrella organisation representing more than 300 member organisations across 99 countries, conducted a global survey to assess the effects of COVID-19 on viral hepatitis services and people living with viral hepatitis [52]. According to their statistics, only 47 of all 132 (36 per cent) respondents were able to access viral hepatitis testing. One hundred and one respondents provided reasons for their lack of access to testing, with the main one cited as the closure of testing facilities (indicated by 46 respondents). The closure of testing facilities was reported by 16 of 54 (30 per cent) respondents outside the United States. Sixty-six of the 101 (65 per cent) respondents believed another key reason people were not accessing testing was due to COVID-19. Twenty-three of 68 (34 per cent) respondents outside the United States were unable to access their medications during this time. The lack of access to medications was more common in low- and middle-income countries (LMICs). Only 5 of 64 (8 per cent) respondents from the United States living with viral hepatitis were unable to access treatment during the pandemic. Sixty-four respondents gave reasons for lack of access to treatment, including 32 (50 per cent) who felt that the cause was people avoiding healthcare facilities due to COVID-19 (14 [64 per cent] of 22 in LMICs). A lack of specific information on COVID-19 for people living with viral hepatitis was also a concern. Only 39 of 131 (30 per cent) responses indicated that adequate information on COVID-19 was provided to people living with viral hepatitis in their country [53].

Osteoporosis. As a chronic condition, osteoporosis generally requires sustained medical intervention(s) to limit the risks of additional bone loss, compromised skeletal integrity and fracture occurrence. Further complicating this issue is the abrupt cessation of some therapies, which can be associated with an increased risk of harm. It is in this context that the COVID-19 pandemic has brought unprecedented disruption to the provision of healthcare globally, including near-universal requirements for social distancing [54].

Rare diseases. A study by Ref. [55] in Hong Kong examined the impact of the COVID-19 pandemic on 272 rare disease patients with 89 distinct rare diseases, using a cross-sectional online survey in April 2020 from the patients' and caregivers' perspectives. The pandemic impacted the health status (46 per cent), service use patterns (71 per cent), mental health (79 per cent), daily living (82 per cent), social life (92 per cent) and financial status (81 per cent) of patients. Health status, medical status, rehabilitation and mental health were more impacted by the COVID-19 pandemic in the group of patients with any level of dependency, according to the Barthel Index for Activities of Daily Living, compared with those who were fully independent.

Severe mental illness. Analysis by Tzur Bitan and colleagues suggested that a substantial survival gap persisted between controls and people with schizophrenia throughout the first year of the pandemic [56]. These findings contributed to the growing body of evidence showing severe mental illnesses and psychotic disorders represent a significant and independent risk factor of COVID-19–associated mortality. Ref. [57] reported that the first increased mortality among people with mental disorders emerged in September 2020, about halfway through the follow-up period of this study, but these new insights apparently did not translate to a specific action or better outcomes for these patients. In fact, the mortality gap was found to be larger in the second half of the follow-up window (HR 2·72 late phase versus 2·15 early phase). Hospital admission rates associated with COVID-19 for people with schizophrenia were also found to be higher in Israel. This finding has been replicated in other studies, although more equivocally, possibly reflecting country differences in healthcare organisations and patients' access to care [56].

People with chronic diseases are at increased risk of severe illness from COVID-19 and vulnerable to the potential worsening of pre-existing conditions because of disruptions to their care. Ref. [58] analysed the evidence on chronic disease management from Australia, Belgium and the Netherlands and identified lessons that could be instructive in the Australian context, as outlined here:

1. telehealth services to support chronic disease management. It is important to ensure patients who are disadvantaged by the digital divide are still able to access care in ways that keep them and others safe.

2. self-management support that requires well-resourced and supported teams. Patients need continued support and encouragement from their primary care team to stay on track to manage their chronic conditions, especially those who are vulnerable and may be isolated during periods of extended lockdown.

3. proactive care that benefits patients and mitigates risk. Electronic medical records have been valuable for identifying and contacting vulnerable patients who need close monitoring. It is important to engage with patients before any escalation of their condition to mitigate risk.

4. community partnerships that offer opportunities for innovation. Maintaining and enhancing linkages between acute and community sectors has been important in ensuring continuity of chronic disease management during the COVID-19 pandemic, especially in low resource settings.

5. consideration of funding model reform. The anticipated increase in chronic conditions and complications, especially among individuals who have experienced delays in diagnosis and treatment, makes a focus on funding model reform all the more urgent to consider, particularly in regions where disruptions to healthcare services have been substantial.

2.3.2 Conclusion

In this section, we investigated the impacts of COVID-19 on patients with high-incidence chronic diseases. The impact of COVID-19 on people with or at risk for chronic disease cannot be overstated. COVID-19 has impeded chronic disease prevention and disrupted disease management [59]. COVID-19 patients presented with hypertension, diabetes, and coronary heart diseases are more likely to progress to severe conditions. COVID-19 patients with cardiovascular diseases are associated with a higher risk of mortality. Chronic diseases like HIV, diabetes, and kidney diseases are immunosuppressing cases, making patients more vulnerable to infections. These patients with COVID-19 are less likely to be cured. COVID-19 is one of the leading causes of heart disease and is responsible for about 5% of the cases of acute heart failure [60].

2.4 IMPACT ON PATIENTS WITH CANCER

Cancer patients have been experiencing extra challenges during the COVID-19 pandemic. Those with compromised immune systems or pre-existing medical conditions may be at increased risk of contracting COVID-19 and more severe infections. Meanwhile, due to the reduced number of general medical services, some cancer patients have delayed their visits to clinicians and pathology testing. Cancer Australia [10] investigated MBS claims to understand the impact of COVID-19 on cancer patients' medical services and procedures in Australia. The analyses showed national reductions in the total monthly services for diagnostic and therapeutic procedures during the initial COVID-19 period between March and May 2020, including procedures related to breast, colorectal, lung, prostate and skin cancers. These decreases occurred between March and April 2020, and for some procedure groups, decreases were more pronounced in April and May 2020.

2.4.1 Literature Review

Bladder cancer. Most bladder cancer patients have been affected by delayed diagnosis and therapy during the COVID-19 pandemic. Ref. [61] reported that the fatality rate of bladder cancer overweighed COVID-19 by far and could be as high as 52 per cent. The paper proposed a new way to perform the screening and monitoring of bladder cancer by taking into consideration the aggressiveness and capacity to progress depending on its stage. Ref. [62] concluded that increased fatality rates resulted from delayed cancer diagnoses and management during the pandemic. Delayed diagnoses and management led to the risk that many thousands of bladder cancer cases were going undetected and untreated, causing a surge in untreated incidences during the pandemic. This surge in advanced bladder cancer was in addition to the knock-on effects (rise in demand for cancer-related services once the pandemic has passed).

Breast cancer. Delayed diagnosis and therapy have also occurred for breast cancer patients. Ref. [63] reported that there were delays in many aspects of breast cancer care, including routine clinical visits (32 per cent), surveillance imaging (14 per cent), routine mammograms (11 per cent), reconstructions (10 per cent), radiation therapy (5 per cent), hormonal therapy (5 per cent), mastectomies (5 per cent) and chemotherapy (4 per cent). About 30 per cent reported no delays. About 30 per cent reported they chose or considered delaying or changing their own treatment plans due to concerns about contracting COVID-19. About 11 per cent reported that COVID-19 affected their desire or ability to seek a second opinion. In addition, it was also suggested that the following breast cancer treatments can weaken the immune system:

- all standard chemotherapy drugs, such as Taxol (chemical name: paclitaxel), Taxotere (chemical name: docetaxel), Cytoxan (chemical name: cyclophosphamide) and carboplatin

- certain targeted therapies, such as Ibrance (chemical name: palbociclib), Kisqali (chemical name: ribociclib), Verzenio (chemical name: abemaciclib) and Piqray (chemical name: alpelisib)

If patients had received these treatments in the past, it is not clear if they are at higher risk of developing serious complications from COVID-19.

Colon and rectal cancer. COVID-19's impacts on colon and rectal cancer (CRC) patients have been limited. Ref. [64] reported that, during the pandemic, outpatient volumes decreased significantly, especially those of non-local and elderly patients, whereas the number of chemotherapies and surgeries remained the same. About 710 CRC patients underwent curative resection. The proportion of patients who received laparoscopic surgeries was 49.4 per cent, significantly higher than the 39.5 per cent during the same period in 2019. The proportion of major complications during the pandemic was not significantly different from the control group. The mean hospital stay was significantly longer than the control group. This suggested that CRC patients confirmed to be infection free can receive routine treatment. Using online medical counselling and appropriate identification, treatment and follow-up can be effectively maintained. Adjuvant and palliative chemotherapy should not be discontinued. Endoscopic polypectomy, elective, palliative and multidisciplinary surgeries can be postponed, while curative surgery should proceed as usual. For elderly CRC patients, endoscopic surgery and neoadjuvant radiotherapy are recommended. Ref. [65] showed that the prevalence of COVID-19 infection was 45.1 per cent in CRC patients. This demonstrates a high COVID-19 infection rate among these patients, but there is no a significant correlation for COVID-19 infection in CRC patients across the global population.

Kidney cancer (renal cell and renal pelvis). Kidney cancer is cancer starting in the cells of the kidney. The most common type of kidney cancer is renal cell carcinoma (RCC), accounting for about 90 per cent of all cases [66]. COVID-19's impacts on the mortality of kidney cancer patients have not been conclusive. Ref. [67] reported that the overall mortality of COVID-19 patients with kidney cancer was lower (11.8 per cent) than those with other malignancies. However, the Thoracic Cancers International COVID-19 Collaboration (TERAVOLT) international registry of patients with thoracic tumours and French and Spanish registries demonstrated a higher mortality rate (14.6–34.6 per cent) and hospitalisation rate for these patients (72.4–76 per cent).

Leukaemia Leukaemia is a broad term for cancers of the blood cells. The type of leukaemia depends on the blood cell that becomes cancerous and whether it grows quickly or slowly [68]. Ref [69] convincingly demonstrated that COVID-19 may result in fatal complications for patients with different kinds of leukaemia. Due to the combined effect of disease and treatment-related immunodeficiency, patients with haematological malignancies may be at high risk of developing severe disease if infected by COVID-19. Patients with chronic lymphocytic leukaemia (CLL) may be particularly vulnerable. Two early international surveys reported that more than one-third of CLL patients had a fatal outcome if hospitalised due to COVID-19.

However, these reports included patients from various sources and were identified at the very beginning of the pandemic. Less severe cases were not included.

Liver and bile duct cancer. The COVID-19 pandemic has posed unprecedented challenges to healthcare systems, and it may have heavily impacted patients with liver cancer. Liver cancer patients appear to be at higher risk of mortality, especially those who have undergone surgery or received a systemic treatment in the previous month. Liver cancer patients are a highly vulnerable category. These patients are often older, have multiple comorbidities and in most cases suffer from an underlying liver disease, which is responsible for a baseline dysfunction of both innate and adaptive immune responses [70]. Ref. [71] evaluated whether the schedules of liver cancer screening or procedures were interrupted or delayed due to the COVID-19 pandemic. The study found that the first wave of the COVID-19 pandemic had a tremendous impact on the routine care of patients with liver cancer. Modifications in screening, diagnostic and treatment algorithms may have also significantly impaired outcomes for these patients.

Lung cancer (including bronchus). A substantial number of patients infected with COVID-19 develop acute respiratory distress syndrome and need advanced healthcare facilities, including invasive mechanical ventilation [72]. This paper studied the effect of COVID-19 on the immune system, ground glass opacity (GGO) and potential neoplastic changes in the lungs due to COVID-19 infection. However, there have still been challenges in lung cancer therapy during the COVID-19 pandemic due to similarities between lung cancer progression and COVID-19 [73]. This has posed a major challenge to clinicians in distinguishing lung cancer evolution from a potential COVID-19 super-infection based on radiological and clinical evidence. Importantly, these specific conditions require very different therapeutic approaches. Ref. [74] presented a practical multidisciplinary and international overview to assist in the treatment of lung cancer patients during the pandemic, with the caveat that evidence was lacking in many areas. Ref. [75] reported that COVID-19 was severe in patients with lung cancer (62 per cent hospitalised and 25 per cent died). Although severe, COVID-19 has accounted for a minority of overall lung cancer deaths during the pandemic (11 per cent overall). This paper found that cancer-specific features, including prior thoracic surgery/radiation and recent systemic therapies, did not impact severity. Among hospitalised patients, hydroxychloroquine did not improve COVID-19 outcomes.

Melanoma. Due to the COVID-19 pandemic, planned medical and surgical activities have been postponed. For the dermatology community, this interruption to the healthcare system has led to delays in the diagnosis and treatment of melanoma. Neglecting melanoma can result in increased mortality, morbidity and healthcare costs [76]. For melanoma patients, based on the current considerations of the major oncologic societies and the clinical practice, Ref. [77] suggested:

encouraging patients not to discontinue ongoing target therapy or immunotherapy independently,

in case of flu symptoms, patients should not discontinue therapy but immediately contact their oncologist or dermato-oncologist,

performing a swab before starting or continuing medical chemotherapy/immunotherapy or, in the case of major surgeries, requiring frequent attendance at a hospital, and

in the case of COVID-19–positive (symptomatic or paucisymptomatic) patients, the paper suggested evaluating patients on a case-by-case basis and, if necessary, suspending a cycle of treatment for both treatments.

Non-Hodgkin's lymphoma. Patients diagnosed with B-cell non-Hodgkin's lymphoma (B-NHL), particularly if recently treated with anti-CD20 antibodies, are at risk of severe COVID-19 [78]. Prolonged COVID-19 is an emerging issue for patients with lymphoma or immune deficiency. Ref. [79] examined the prolonged length of in-hospital stays due to COVID-19 among patients with lymphoma to assess its determinants and outcomes. The findings of Ref. [79] may contribute to the management of lymphoma during the pandemic and support evaluating specific therapeutic approaches and exploring questions on the efficacy and timing of vaccinations for this particular population.

Pancreatic cancer. As the COVID-19 pandemic had an important impact on pancreatic cancer surgeries, Ref. [80] examined guidelines for the prompt intervention and prevention of the spread of viral infections in surgical environments during the pandemic. The paper suggested that high-volume centres for pancreatic surgery should be preferred and their activity maintained. Telemedicine has proven to be efficient during the pandemic and should be implemented in the near future. Ref. [81] suggested using neoadjuvant treatment and conducting safe surgeries while protecting patients in a controlled environment to improve oncological outcomes. They may also delay high-risk, resource-intensive pancreatectomies while hospitals redirect valuable resources to address surging COVID-19 cases in their communities. Even an optimal oncologic procedure performed in a hazardous setting could shorten patient survival if recovery is complicated by factors such as COVID-19 infection. Ref. [82] suggested optimising outcomes for patients with pancreatic cancer. It is vital that these decisions be individualised for patients following multidisciplinary team discussions and that comprehensive counselling on treatment options be available prior to providing informed consent for treatment.

Prostate cancer. Ref. [83] provided recommendations for prostate cancer management during the pandemic through general considerations, diagnostic procedures, different disease stages, treatment modules, patient support and interdisciplinary collaboration. The overall goal is to minimise the risk of infection while avoiding unnecessary delays and compromises in managing outcomes. Practical issues during the pandemic are addressed, such as the use of invasive diagnostic procedures, robotic-assisted laparoscopic prostatectomy, hypofractionated radiotherapy and prolonged androgen deprivation therapy. Ref. [84] provided suggestions for managing patients with prostate cancer during the COVID-19 pandemic. They adopted some actions learned from the experiences of different centres in the United States (New York) and other countries (Italy, Spain, France, India, Germany, England, Belgium and Russia) during online webinars and urologic meetings. They suggested managing patients with prostate cancer at the beginning of the COVID-19 pandemic by changing office routines, stratifying patients according to the National Comprehensive Cancer Network (NCCN) risk profile and adopting COVID-19–based criteria to select patients for surgery. These are necessary actions for maintaining best-quality treatment and minimising viral infections among oncological patients. Robot-assisted radical prostatectomy (RARP) during the COVID-19 pandemic proved safe and feasible for patients and healthcare workers when the necessary precautions described in the article were undertaken.

Thyroid cancer. Most patients with thyroid nodules and thyroid cancer referred for diagnostic checks and treatment have not been considered at higher risk of infection from COVID-19 compared with the general population [85]. There have been several significant impacts on treatment and diagnosis. First, diagnosis has been delayed due to social isolation, reduced access to investigations and staff redeployment. Second, treatment planning has needed to take into account the risk of nosocomial transmission of the virus to patients and/or staff. Third, there are some specific concerns with interactions between the virus, its treatments and cancer [86–89].

Skin cancer. The effect of skin cancer on the risk of adverse outcomes from COVID-19 remains unknown [90]. Few studies have shown that patients with cancer and COVID-19 have higher rates of mortality and hospitalisations than those without cancer, perhaps due to a combination of delayed diagnosis and pre-existing comorbidities from chemotherapy and radiation treatments [91]. However, some studies have suggested that cancer may be protective against mortality from COVID-19, possibly from natural immunosuppression reducing the negative effects of a cytokine storm [92].

The main effect of the COVID-19 pandemic on skin cancer was reducing diagnosis numbers. Research based on the Northern Cancer Network data in the United Kingdom [93] compared the COVID-19 era (from 23 March 2020 to 23 June 2020) with the same period in 2019 (pre–COVID-19). In the COVID-19 period, there was a decrease of 68.6 per cent in skin cancer diagnoses. Interestingly, skin cancer waiting times were also reduced in the COVID-19 period compared with the pre-COVID-19 period (median of 8 and 12 days, respectively). Besides reduced diagnosis numbers, the core challenge has been to achieve the best possible balance between the risk of cancer progression and infectious disease [94].

2.4.2 Conclusion

In this section, we investigated the impacts of COVID-19 on the most common cancer types listed in Ref. [95]. For cancer patients who require immunotherapy, the work focuses on complications and mortality due to COVID-19. As these patients are more vulnerable to the virus, increased risks of compromised immune systems are an overriding factor for creating treatment plans. For cancer patients requiring hospitalisation or surgery, there are concerns about the risks of COVID-19 to both patients and health workers. A variety of published articles have provided suggestions on whether the services should be delayed or carried out as normal. Additionally, surrogate healthcare guidelines for delayed services are discussed.

2.5 IMPACT ON PATIENTS WITH END-OF-LIFE/ PALLIATIVE CARE

2.5.1 Literature Review

The COVID-19 pandemic has caused over three million deaths globally and over 900 in Australia [96]. Healthcare providers have been faced with difficult ethical decisions of prioritising ICU care and ventilator support for patients with higher chances of survival. Thus, the COVID-19 pandemic has disrupted the last days of life of patients receiving end-of-life-care. Palliative care [97] is a complex interaction between patients and caregivers. It is more likely to have been impacted by the COVID-19 pandemic.

2.5.2 Pain Management

Chronic pain is the leading cause of disability in the world. It is associated with multiple psychiatric comorbidities and has been causally linked to the opioid crisis. Access to pain treatment has been called a fundamental human right by numerous organisations. The current COVID-19 pandemic has led to strained medical resources, which has created a dilemma for physicians charged with limiting the spread of the contagion and treating patients [98]. From a societal perspective, chronic pain not only leads to suffering but also impairs daily activities and increases illicit drug consumption, sick leave frequency and disability and pension payments. This leads to high downstream societal costs. It also poses a major problem for public health and creates substantial costs for healthcare systems and disability insurance [99,100].

To help patients overcome shortages and/or interruptions to pain management services during the COVID-19 pandemic, a series of instructive articles was published, providing value experience and suggestions. Ref. [101] summed up their lessons and pain management strategies at the beginning of the pandemic. For example, in terms of lessons learned, they recommended:

1. keeping information transparent and up to date and taking action quickly and firmly,

2. quarantine and personal protection,

3. telemedicine support and

4. pain management for patients with and without COVID-19.

In relation to pain management strategies, they recommended:

1. outpatient and inpatient pain management,

2. telemedicine support and patient home visits and

3. special case reports for patients with and without COVID-19.

Ref. [46] discussed four related factors to help guide healthcare professionals caring for patients with chronic pain and provide guidance for those attempting to rapidly transition to remote care with technology. The authors also discussed lessons for the future of pain treatment centres. The four related factors are:

1. the public health consequences of COVID-19 for patients with pain,

2. the consequences of not treating these patients during the pandemic,

3. options for remote assessment and management and

4. clinical evidence supporting remote therapies.

Ref. [102] analysed the impact of the COVID-19 pandemic on chronic pain treatment and addressed the types of strategies that can be implemented or supported to overcome the imposed limitations in the delivery of chronic pain patient care. They provided a series of recommendations for the best practice management of pain management patients, as outlined here:

1. infection control in healthcare settings according to the Centers for Disease Control (CDC) recommendations, namely body temperature checks, social distancing, hand hygiene, face masks and gloves during patient care and cleaning for the patient care environment;

2. triaging the risks of COVID-19 screening patients and personnel for symptoms of COVID-19;

3. triaging pain procedures in elective, urgent and emergent situations, that is, suspending elective cases, proceeding with emergent ones and considering case by case in urgent situations;

4. suspending in-person visits whenever possible; in-person visits remain an option that should be taken into consideration according to several factors, such as acuity and severity of pain, whether the patient has a comorbid psychiatric condition, occupational considerations (such as whether the patient is also a caregiver or has children), the likelihood of the visit/procedure providing meaningful benefit, the likelihood of the patient seeking emergency services or starting opioids and the need for physical examination;

5. adapting ongoing therapy to reduce the risk of COVID-19;

6. performing urgent procedures with a minimal number of personnel, ideally by a single physician, and avoiding deep sedation requiring airway support; and

7. considering intrathecal pump refills as an emergent interventional pain procedure; in some cases, in-home pump refills can be planned.

Ref. [98] provided a framework for pain practitioners and institutions to balance the conflicting goals of risk mitigation for healthcare providers and patients, the conservation of resources and access to pain management services. Factors that should be taken into consideration when deciding whether to see a patient in person, change the appointment to telemedicine, postpone the visit or perform a procedure include

- acuity

- comorbid psychiatric (e.g., severe pain-related depression) and social (e.g., single mother of young children with limited resources) considerations

- pain level and accompanying functional impairment

- likelihood of the visit/procedure providing meaningful benefit

- likelihood of the patient seeking scarce emergency services or starting opioids

- need for physical examination

- risk associated with an in-person visit or procedure

- work status (e.g., whether the patient is currently working or likely to return to work with adequate pain treatment)

- job (i.e., prioritising first responders and other critical personnel who will provide the greatest benefit to society)

2.5.3 Palliative Care

Palliative care has played a central role in a healthcare institutions' responses to the COVID-19 pandemic [103]. The high numbers of critically ill and dying patients created a sharp increase in the need for the expert management of dyspnoea, delirium and serious illness conversations [104]. During the pandemic in LMIC countries, the needs of people seeking palliative care services were likely to be more severe than those in high-income countries [105]. The burden was caused by various aspects, including poor healthcare systems and outbreak preparedness, severe shortages in personal protective equipment and medical technology, challenges in enforcing physical distancing regulations and reliance on informal employment. In such settings, patients with severe COVID-19 unable to access the limited supply of intensive care resources or hospital beds are expected to suffer and die at home. They would be cared for by family members without personal protective equipment and access to relevant information, training or palliative care resources. These caregivers will probably become infected and spread the disease [106–108].

The delivery of palliative care has brought economic benefits during the pandemic. It has been found to be less costly than the usual care comparators. It has also reduced the burden on health systems, which has benefited other patients. Compared with formal care treatments, it improves both the quality of end-of-life care and dying [106,107,109]. Changes in palliative care delivery during the pandemic are threefold. First, telemedicine has greatly developed during the COVID-19 pandemic. Second, the regulations have been changed to better coordinate the delivery of palliative care and quarantine orders to ensure physical distancing. Third, family members have participated more in palliative care during the pandemic because of the overwhelming strain on the healthcare system [110].

Ref. [100] is a guide to understanding of the scope of challenges that a pandemic or disaster poses for the delivery of health services, including palliative care. It describes the role of palliative care in supporting different patient journeys during COVID-19, including the importance of advance care planning, the ethical challenges and distress that may arise around resource allocation or rationing decisions should they become necessary, the overarching principles that govern the distribution of finite resources and the practical realities of how such principles are implemented. It invites governments—commonwealth, state and territory—to take the lead in working with clinicians and communities through open and transparent processes to create the necessary guidelines for decision-making during a disaster or pandemic. Finally, it describes the role of governments in accepting legal and moral responsibility for guidelines that instruct difficult binary choices of treatment refusal when resources cannot meet demand during a major disaster, severe epidemic or pandemic such as COVID-19.

Many studies have investigated the clinical characteristics, end-of-life care, symptomatology and use of supportive therapies in consecutively admitted patients who died from COVID-19. Ref. [111] was one of the first and largest Australian reports on the end of life and symptom experience of people dying from COVID-19 in a large Victorian tertiary hospital. This information should help clinicians anticipate the palliative care needs of these patients; for example, recognising that higher starting doses of opioids and sedatives may help reduce the prevalence and severity of breathlessness and agitation near death. Ref. [112] undertook a case series of 101 patients with COVID-19 referred for hospital palliative care in the United Kingdom. The paper identified their symptom burden, management and responses to treatment and outcomes.

Ref. [113] explored the effects of the pandemic on the experiences of next-of-kin and carers who encountered the death of a loved one in residential aged care facilities (RACFs). The study identified the many COVID-19 pandemic-related challenges faced by the participants and their dying loved ones in RACFs. Access to palliative care and bereavement support is crucial for dying residents and for the grieving, and it has been made more difficult by the pandemic.

Ref. [114] described an innovative social work and nursing approach to brokering patient and family care amid social distancing and the visit restrictions of COVID-19. They began with a description of the setting, the inter-professional palliative medicine team and the humanistic patient and family interventions employed to build trust and connection and foster hope. They presented a qualitative synthesis of the interdisciplinary palliative medicine team's journal reflections on barriers to patient and family care during COVID-19. It also explored patients' and families' reactions to the team's humanistic interventions and insights into the team members' personal and professional meaning explorations during the pandemic.

Ref. [115] provided information to help understand and create advance care planning for Australians during the COVID-19 pandemic. Ref. [116] described the challenges that UK specialist palliative care services experienced regarding advance care planning during the COVID-19 pandemic and the changes they made to support timely conversations. The authors suggested that professionals and healthcare providers need to ensure advance care planning is individualised by tailoring it to the values, priorities and ethnic/cultural/religious contexts of each person. Policymakers need to consider how high-quality advance care planning can be resourced as a part of standard healthcare ahead of future pandemic waves. To facilitate this, questions must be proposed for consideration at each level of the social ecological model.

2.5.4 Conclusion

In this section, we investigated the impacts of COVID-19 on pain management and palliative care. Chronic pain management during COVID-19 pandemic has been a challenging process, especially with the growing evidence that COVID-19 infection is associated with myalgias, referred pain and widespread hyperalgesia [117]. Palliative care is an approach that improves the quality of life of patients and their families facing the problems associated with life-limiting illnesses through the prevention and relief of suffering by means of early identification and impeccable assessment and treatment of pain and other problems, physical, psychosocial and spiritual [118]. As health systems have become strained under COVID-19, providing safe and effective palliative care, including end-of-life care, has become especially vital and especially difficult [100].

2.6 ANALYSIS METHODOLOGY

To analyse the impact of the COVID-19 pandemic on chronic diseases and cancers, the analysis team followed these steps:

- identifying analysis questions

- preparing and pre-processing available datasets

- conducting analysis

Identify analysis questions. Key analytic questions are outlined in the following.

- identifying change categories (e.g., dispensing patterns for drugs, surgery, radiotherapy, hospitalisations and use of telehealth), which were the initial input features for conducting the analysis, compared with those cohorts without COVID-19

- identifying health outcomes for chronic diseases (e.g., death, complications/adverse events, disease progression and healthcare service pathways), which were considered the targets of the analysis

- identifying health outcomes for cancers (e.g., prescribing of anti-depressants, changes in chronic disease management plans for cancer patients, shifts in palliative care from hospital to home, remoteness, access to specialists, uptake of diagnostic testing and monitoring, hospitalisations, complications/adverse events and death)

- analysing correlations between changes and outcomes.

Data pre-processing. The healthcare activities of people with chronic conditions mainly consisted of prescriptions, visiting doctors [119], and hospitalisation (ICD-10). Key data pre-processing steps are outlined in the following:

- the linkage between those available datasets was the first step in conducting analysis in this task

TABLE 2.1   Typical Chronic Diseases and Cancer—Code Mapping

Diseases	Anatomical Therapeutic Chemical (ATC) Classification	International Classification of Diseases (ICD)-10
Diabetes	A10	E10–E14
Kidney Disease	B03XA01, B03XA02, B03XA03, B03AE02, B03AE03, B03AE05	N18
Poorly Controlled Blood Pressure	C02, C03AA, C07, C08, C09	I10, R03
HIV	J05AE, J05AR, J05AF, J05AG, J05AX07, J05AX09, J05AJ	B20–B24
Hepatitis	J07CA09, J07CA11, J07CA13, J07CA05, J07CA07, J07CA12, J07CA08, J06BB11, J07BC02, J06BB04, J07BC01, J07CA10	B15–B19
Osteoporosis		M80–M82
Cancer	L01	C81–C96, D693, Z511, Z510

- extracting data of people with typical chronic diseases (e.g., diabetes, kidney disease, poorly controlled blood pressure, HIV, hepatitis, and osteoporosis) from the linked data
- extracting data of people with cancer and processing each individual's data according to a sequence of activities with timestamps
- generating disease-code mapping (Table. 2.1).

Data analysis on typical chronic diseases and cancer. Key data analytic activities are outlined in the following:

- statistical analysis on patient cohorts, such as certain demographics, diagnosis profiles or healthcare utilisation patterns and health outcomes
- analysing how health and social outcomes and the utilisation of reproductive health and fertility services have changed during COVID-19

- analysing the impact on specialist clinics that provide services for patients with chronic conditions

- analysing correlations between learned patient pathways and outcomes

- analysing risk factors for poor health outcomes before and after the COVID-19 pandemic.

2.7 CONCLUSION

This chapter reviewed literature from academic research journals and government health organisation reports conducted on how COVID-19 impacted patients with complex health conditions. We investigated COVID-19 impact on three vulnerable cohorts categorised in this review, such as patients with chronic disease, patients with cancer and patients with end-of-life care. Analysis methodology and a typical chronic disease and cancer code mapping table were proposed in this chapter to identify each cohort from an analytics perspective. The chapter presents a comprehensive literature review on the COVID-19 impact on patients with health conditions. This chapter provided evidence on how to improve the quality of life for vulnerable populations and to inform a national response strategy for future pandemics, which seem inevitable in a highly globalised economy. The chapter presents a comprehensive literature review on the COVID-19 impact on patients with health conditions. Data-driven analysis of the impact of the pandemic on patients with complex health conditions helps governments change national response strategies according to real-world impacts. The actionable knowledge and management discovered by this literature review can support clinical actions and aid decision-making for diagnosis and treatment of diseases in real environments. The proposed analysis methodology and typical chronic disease and cancer code mapping table can be implemented in the healthcare domain to improve decision-making.

ACKNOWLEDGEMENTS

This work is supported by the Australian Government Department of Health and Aged Care (the Health). We thank Paul Martin from the Health for his careful reading of the manuscript and his many insightful comments and suggestions.

REFERENCES

1. Hongzhou Lu, Charles W Stratton, and Yi Wei Tang. Outbreak of pneumonia of unknown etiology in Wuhan, China: The mystery and the miracle. Journal of Medical Virology, 92(4):401, 2020.
2. World Health Organization and Statement on the Second Meeting of the International Health Regulations (2005) Emergency Committee regarding the outbreak of novel coronavirus (2019-ncov). www.who.int/news/item/30-01-2020-statement-on-the-second-meeting-of-the-international-health-regulations-(2005)-emergency-committee-regarding-the-outbreak-of-novel-coronavirus-(2019-ncov), 2020. Accessed 14 October 2021.
3. World Health Organization. WHO coronavirus (COVID-19) dashboard. https://covid19.who.int/, 2020. Accessed 14 October 2021.
4. International Labour Organization. ILO Monitor: COVID-19 and the World of Work. Seventh edition. Updated estimates and analysis. Geneva: International Labour Organization, pp. 1–35, 2021.
5. Australian Institute of Health and Welfare. AIHW-COVID-19 impact. www.aihw.gov.au/COVID-19, 2021. Accessed 14 October 2021.
6. Australian Government Department of Health. Coronavirus (COVID-19) case numbers and statistics. www.health.gov.au/news/health-alerts/novel-coronavirus-2019-ncov-health-alert/coronavirus-COVID-19-case-numbers-and-statistics, 2021. Accessed 14 October 2021.
7. Australian Government Department of Treasury. National plan to transition to Australia's national COVID-19 response economic impact analysis. https://treasury.gov.au/publication/p2021-196731, 2021. Accessed 14 October 2021.
8. Australian Bureau of Statistics. Coronavirus (COVID-19) case numbers and statistics. www.abs.gov.au/COVID-19, 2021. Accessed 14 October 2021.
9. Australian Bureau of Statistics. Multi-Agency Data Integration Project (MADIP). www.abs.gov.au/about/data-services/data-integration/integrated-data/multi-agency-data-integration-project-madip, 2021. Accessed 26 November 2021.
10. Cancer Australia. National and Jurisdictional Data on the Impact of COVID-19 on Medical Services and Procedures in Australia: Breast, Colorectal, Lung, Prostate and Skin Cancers. Surry Hills: Cancer Australia Sydney, pp. 1–64, 2020.
11. Our World in Data. Stringency index. https://ourworldindata.org/covid-stringency-index, 2021. Accessed 14 October 2021.
12. The Oxford COVID-19 Government Response Tracker. COVID-19 government response tracker. www.bsg.ox.ac.uk/research/research-projects/COVID-19-government-response-tracker, 2021. Accessed 14 October 2021.
13. Spectator Australia. If this is a global pandemic, why aren't we loosening our chains like the rest of the world? H-this-is-a-global-pandemic-why-arent-we-loosening-our-chains-like-the-rest-of-the-world/, 2021. Accessed 14 October 2021.

14. Australian Bureau of Statistics. State economies and the stringency of COVID-19 containment measures. www.abs.gov.au/articles/state-econo mies-and-stringency-COVID-19-containment-measures, 2020. Accessed 14 October 2021.
15. Australian Institute of Health and Welfare. Australia's health 2020. www. aihw.gov.au/reports-data/australias-health, 2020. Accessed 15 February 2022.
16. Kevin J Clerkin, Justin A Fried, Jayant Raikhelkar, et al. COVID-19 and cardiovascular disease. Circulation, 141(20):1648–1655, 2020.
17. Ajit Magadum and Raj Kishore. Cardiovascular manifestations of COVID-19 infection. Cells, 9(11):2508, 2020.
18. Tommaso Gori, Jos Lelieveld, and Thomas Münzel. Perspective: Cardiovascular disease and the COVID-19 pandemic. Basic Research in Cardiology, 115(3):1–4, 2020.
19. Awadhesh Kumar Singh, Ritesh Gupta, Amerta Ghosh, and Anoop Misra. Diabetes in COVID-19: Prevalence, pathophysiology, prognosis and practical considerations. Diabetes & Metabolic Syndrome: Clinical Research & Reviews, 14(4):303–310, 2020.
20. Ad'ele Lasbleiz, Bertrand Cariou, Patrice Darmon, et al. Phenotypic characteristics and development of a hospitalization prediction risk score for outpatients with diabetes and COVID-19: The DIABCOVID study. Journal of Clinical Medicine, 9(11):3726, 2020.
21. Ranganath Muniyappa and Sriram Gubbi. COVID-19 pandemic, coronaviruses, and diabetes mellitus. American Journal of Physiology-Endocrinology and Metabolism, 318(5):E736–E741, 2020.
22. Ritesh Gupta, Amerta Ghosh, Awadhesh Kumar Singh, and Anoop Misra. Clinical considerations for patients with diabetes in times of COVID-19 epidemic. Diabetes & Metabolic Syndrome, 14(3):211, 2020.
23. Zhen Li, Ming Wu, Jiwei Yao, et al. Caution on kidney dysfunctions of COVID-19 patients. medRxiv, pp. 1–25, 2020.
24. Paul Gabarre, Guillaume Dumas, Thibault Dupont, et al. Acute kidney injury in critically ill patients with COVID-19. Intensive Care Medicine, 46(7):1339–1348, 2020.
25. Sachin J Shah, Peter N Barish, Priya A Prasad, et al. Clinical features, diagnostics, and outcomes of patients presenting with acute respiratory illness: A retrospective cohort study of patients with and without COVID-19. eClinicalMedicine, 27:100518, 2020.
26. Chiara Masetti, Elena Generali, Francesca Colapietro, et al. High mortality in COVID-19 patients with mild respiratory disease. European Journal of Clinical Investigation, 50(9):e13314, 2020.
27. Glenis K Scadding, Peter W Hellings, Claus Bachert, et al. Allergic respiratory disease care in the COVID-19 era: A EUFOREA statement. The World Allergy Organization Journal, 13(5), 2020.
28. Chih Cheng Lai, Wen Chien Ko, Ping Ing Lee, et al. Extra-respiratory manifestations of COVID-19. International Journal of Antimicrobial Agents, 56(2):106024, 2020.

29. World Health Organization. Epilepsy. www.who.int/news-room/fact-sheets/detail/epilepsy, 2022. Accessed 14 March 2022.

30. Naoto Kuroda. Epilepsy and COVID-19: Associations and important considerations. Epilepsy & Behavior, 108, 2020.

31. Naoto Kuroda. Epilepsy and COVID-19: Updated evidence and narrative review. Epilepsy & Behavior, 116:107785, 2021.

32. Xiaoting Hao, Dong Zhou, Zhe Li, et al. Severe psychological distress among patients with epilepsy during the COVID-19 outbreak in southwest China. Epilepsia, 61(6):1166–1173, 2020.

33. Elena Fonseca, Manuel Quintana, Sofía Lallana, et al. Epilepsy in time of COVID-19: A survey-based study. Acta Neurologica Scandinavica, 142(6):545–554, 2020.

34. Multiple Sclerosis Limited. Understanding multiple sclerosis. www.ms.org.au/what-is-multiple-sclerosis/understanding-multiple-sclerosis.aspx, 2022. Accessed 16 February 2022.

35. Konrad Rejdak and Pawewl Grieb. Adamantanes might be protective from COVID-19 in patients with neurological diseases: Multiple sclerosis, parkinsonism and cognitive impairment. Multiple Sclerosis and Related Disorders, 42:102163, 2020.

36. Wallace Brownlee, Dennis Bourdette, Simon Broadley, et al. Treating multiple sclerosis and neuromyelitis optica spectrum disorder during the COVID-19 pandemic. Neurology, 94(22):949–952, 2020.

37. Maria Pia Sormani. An Italian programme for COVID-19 infection in multiple sclerosis. The Lancet Neurology, 19(6):481–482, 2020.

38. Centers for Disease Control and Prevention. Common eye disorders and diseases. www.cdc.gov/visionhealth/basics/ced/index.html#::text=external%20icon,Cataract,loss%20in%20the%20United%20States., 2020. Accessed 14 March 2022.

39. Mutasem Elfalah, Saif Aldeen AlRyalat, Mario Damiano Toro, et al. Delayed intravitreal anti-VEGF therapy for patients during the COVID-19 lockdown: An ethical endeavor. Clinical Ophthalmology (Auckland, NZ), 15:661, 2021.

40. Matt J Boyd, Daniel AR Scott, David M Squirrell, and Graham A Wilson. Proof-of-concept calculations to determine the health-adjusted life-year trade-off between intravitreal anti-VEGF injections and transmission of COVID-19. Clinical & Experimental Ophthalmology, 48(9):1276–1285, 2020.

41. April Jorge, Kristin M D'Silva, Andrew Cohen, et al. Temporal trends in severe COVID-19 outcomes in patients with rheumatic disease: A cohort study. The Lancet Rheumatology, 3(2):e131–e137, 2021.

42. Nathaniel P Disser, Andrea J De Micheli, Martin M Schonk, et al. Musculoskeletal consequences of COVID-19. The Journal of Bone & Joint Surgery, 102(14):1197–1204, 2020.

43. Jeffrey R Curtis, Sindhu R Johnson, Donald D Anthony, et al. American College of rheumatology guidance for COVID-19 vaccination in patients with rheumatic and musculoskeletal diseases: Version 2. Arthritis & Rheumatology, 73(8):e30–e45, 2021.

44. Harriet I Kemp, Eve Corner, and Lesley A Colvin. Chronic pain after COVID-19: Implications for rehabilitation. British Journal of Anaesthesia, 125(4):436–440, 2020.

45. Daniel J Clauw, Winfried Häuser, Steven P Cohen, and Mary Ann Fitzcharles. Considering the potential for an increase in chronic pain after the COVID-19 pandemic. Pain, 161(8):1694, 2020.

46. Christopher Eccleston, Fiona M Blyth, Blake F Dear, et al. Managing patients with chronic pain during the COVID-19 outbreak: Considerations for the rapid introduction of remotely supported (eHealth) pain management services. Pain, 161(5):889, 2020.

47. Emanuele Piraccini, Helen Byrne, and Stefania Taddei. Chronic pain management in COVID-19 era. Journal of Clinical Anesthesia, 65:109852, 2020.

48. Roxana Schwab, Katharina Aníc, Kathrin Stewen, et al. Pain experience and social support of endometriosis patients during the COVID-19 pandemic in Germany-results of a web-based cross-sectional survey. PLOS One, 16(8):e0256433, 2021.

49. Mathew Leonardi, Andrew W Horne, Mike Armour, et al. Endometriosis and the Coronavirus (COVID-19) pandemic: Clinical Advice and Future Considerations. Frontiers in Reproductive Health, 2:5, 2020.

50. Hongbo Jiang, Yi Zhou, and Weiming Tang. Maintaining HIV care during the COVID-19 pandemic. The Lancet HIV, 7(5):e308-e309, 2020.

51. Savannah Karmen-Tuohy, Philip M Carlucci, Fainareti N Zervou, et al. Outcomes among HIV-positive patients hospitalized with COVID-19. Journal of Acquired Immune Deficiency Syndromes (1999), 85(1):6–10, 2020.

52. Chris Wingrove, Lucy Ferrier, Cary James, and Su Wang. The impact of COVID-19 on hepatitis elimination. The Lancet Gastroenterology & Hepatology, 5(9):792–794, 2020.

53. Praneet Wander, Marcia Epstein, and David Bernstein. COVID-19 presenting as acute hepatitis. The American Journal of Gastroenterology, 115(6):941–942, 2020.

54. Christian M Girgis and Roderick J Clifton-Bligh. Osteoporosis in the age of COVID-19. Osteoporosis International, 31(7):1189–1191, 2020.

55. Claudia CY Chung, Wilfred HS Wong, Jasmine LF Fung, et al. Impact of COVID-19 pandemic on patients with rare disease in Hong Kong. European Journal of Medical Genetics, 63(12):104062, 2020.

56. Nicole Kozloff, Benoit H Mulsant, Vicky Stergiopoulos, and Aristotle N Voineskos. The COVID-19 global pandemic: Implications for people with schizophrenia and related disorders. Schizophrenia Bulletin, 46(4):752–757, 2020.

57. Livia J De Picker. Closing COVID-19 mortality, vaccination, and evidence gaps for those with severe mental illness. The Lancet Psychiatry, 8(10):854–855, 2021.

58. Anne Parkinson, Sethunya Matenge, Jane Desborough, et al. The impact of COVID-19 on chronic disease management in primary care: Lessons for Australia from the international experience. Medical Journal of Australia, 216(9):445–448, 2022.

59. Karen A Hacker, Peter A Briss, Lisa Richardson, et al. Peer reviewed: Covid-19 and chronic disease: The impact now and in the future. Preventing Chronic Disease, 18, 2021.

60. Ginenus Fekadu, Firomsa Bekele, Tadesse Tolossa, et al. Impact of covid-19 pan-demic on chronic diseases care follow-up and current perspectives in low resource settings: A narrative review. International Journal of Physiology, Pathophysiology and Pharmacology, 13(3):86, 2021.

61. Thiago C Travassos, Joao Marcos Ibrahim De Oliveira, Ivan B Selegatto, and Leonardo O Reis. COVID-19 impact on bladder cancer-orientations for diagnosing, decision making, and treatment. American Journal of Clinical and Experimental Urology, 9(1):132, 2021.

62. Julien Sarkis, Ramy Samaha, Joseph Kattan, and Pierre Sarkis. Bladder cancer during the COVID-19 pandemic: The calm before the storm? Future Science OA, 6(8):FSO615, 2020.

63. Breast Cancer. Special report: COVID-19's impact on breast cancer care. www.breastcancer.org/treatment/COVID-19-and-breast-cancer-care, 2021. Accessed 14 October 2021.

64. Yun Xu, Zong Hao Huang, Charlie Zhi Lin Zheng, et al. The impact of COVID-19 pandemic on colorectal cancer patients: A single-center retrospective study. BMC Gastroenterology, 21(1):1–11, 2021.

65. Mohammad Hossein Antikchi, Hossein Neamatzadeh, Yaser Ghelmani, et al. The risk and prevalence of COVID-19 infection in colorectal cancer patients: A systematic review and meta-analysis. Journal of Gastrointestinal Cancer, 52(1):73–79, 2021.

66. Cancer Council. Kidney cancer. www.cancer.org.au/cancer-information/types-of-cancer/kidney-cancer, 2020. Accessed 8 December 2021.

67. Ilya Tsimafeyeu, Galina Alekseeva, Maria Berkut, et al. COVID-19 in patients with renal cell carcinoma in the Russian Federation. Clinical Genitourinary Cancer, 19(2):e69-e71, 2021.

68. National Institutes of Health. Leukemia. www.cancer.gov/types/leukemia, 2020. Accessed 8 December 2021.

69. Lisa Blixt, Gordana Bogdanovic, Marcus Buggert, et al. COVID-19 in patients with chronic lymphocytic leukemia: Clinical outcome and B-and T-cell immunity during 13 months in consecutive patients. Leukemia, pp. 1–6, 2021.

70. Antonio D'Alessio, Nicola Personeni, Tiziana Pressiani, et al. COVID-19 and liver cancer clinical trials: Not everything is lost. Liver International, 40(7):1541–1544, 2020.

71. Sergio Muñoz-Martínez, Victor Sapena, Alejandro Forner, et al. Assessing the impact of COVID-19 on liver cancer management (CERO-19). JHEP Reports, 3(3):100260, 2021.

72. Pritam Sadhukhan, M Talha Ugurlu, and Mohammad O Hoque. Effect of COVID-19 on lungs: Focusing on prospective malignant phenotypes. Cancers, 12(12):3822, 2020.

73. Luana Calabro, Solange Peters, Jean Charles Soria, et al. Challenges in lung cancer therapy during the COVID-19 pandemic. The Lancet Respiratory Medicine, 8(6):542–544, 2020.

74. Anne Marie C Dingemans, Ross A Soo, Abdul Rahman Jazieh, et al. Treatment guidance for patients with lung cancer during the coronavirus 2019 pandemic. Journal of Thoracic Oncology, 15(7):1119–1136, 2020.

75. Jia Luo, Hira Rizvi, Isabel R Preeshagul, et al. COVID-19 in patients with lung cancer. Annals of Oncology, 31(10):1386–1396, 2020.

76. Tamar Gomolin, Abigail Cline, and Marc Zachary Handler. The danger of neglecting melanoma during the COVID-19 pandemic. Journal of Dermatological Treatment, 31(5):444–445, 2020.

77. Claudio Conforti, Roberta Giuffrida, Nicola Di Meo, and Iris Zalaudek. Management of advanced melanoma in the COVID-19 era. Dermatologic Therapy, 33(4):e13444, 2020.

78. Christopher Perry, Efrat Luttwak, Roi Balaban, et al. Efficacy of the BNT162b2 mRNA COVID-19 vaccine in patients with B-cell non-Hodgkin lymphoma. Blood Advances, 5(16):3053–3061, 2021.

79. Rémy Duléry, Sylvain Lamure, Marc Delord, et al. Prolonged in-hospital stay and higher mortality after COVID-19 among patients with non-Hodgkin lymphoma treated with B-cell depleting immunotherapy. American Journal of Hematology, 96(8):934–944, 2021.

80. Ilaria Pergolini, I Ekin Demir, Christian Stöss, et al. Effects of COVID-19 pandemic on the treatment of pancreatic cancer: A perspective from Central Europe. Digestive Surgery, 38(2):158–165, 2021.

81. Maitham A Moslim, Michael J Hall, Joshua E Meyer, and Sanjay S Reddy. Pancreatic cancer in the era of COVID-19 pandemic: Which one is the lesser of two evils? World Journal of Clinical Oncology, 12(2):54, 2021.

82. Christopher M Jones, Ganesh Radhakrishna, Katharine Aitken, et al. Considerations for the treatment of pancreatic cancer during the COVID-19 pandemic: The UK consensus position. British Journal of Cancer, 123(5):709–713, 2020.

83. Darren Ming Chun Poon, Chi Kwok Chan, Tim Wai Chan, et al. Prostate cancer management in the era of COVID-19: Recommendations from the Hong Kong Urological Association and Hong Kong Society of Uro-oncology. Asia-Pacific Journal of Clinical Oncology, 17:48–54, 2021.

84. Marcio Covas Moschovas, Seetharam Bhat, Travis Rogers, et al. Managing patients with prostate cancer during COVID-19 pandemic: The experience of a high-volume robotic surgery center. Journal of Endourology, 35(3): 305–311, 2021.

85. Alexis Vrachimis, Ioannis Iakovou, Evanthia Giannoula, and Luca Giovanella. Endocrinology in the time of COVID-19: Management of thyroid nodules and cancer. European Journal of Endocrinology, 183(1):G41–G48, 2020.

86. Sohail Bakkar, Khaled Al-Omar, Qusai Aljarrah, et al. Impact of COVID-19 on thyroid cancer surgery and adjunct therapy. Updates in Surgery, 72(3):867–869, 2020.

87. Lorenzo Scappaticcio, Fabían Pitoia, Katherine Esposito, et al. Impact of COVID-19 on the thyroid gland: An update. Reviews in Endocrine and Metabolic Disorders, pp. 1–13, 2020.

88. Anabella Smulever, Erika Abelleira, Fernanda Bueno, and Fabían Pitoia. Thyroid cancer in the era of COVID-19. Endocrine, 70(1):1–5, 2020.

89. Venessa HM Tsang, Matti Gild, Anthony Glover, et al. Thyroid cancer in the age of COVID-19. Endocrine-Related Cancer, 27(11):R407-R416, 2020.

90. Riva Raiker, Haig Pakhchanian, Ali Hussain, and Mei Deng. Outcomes of COVID-19 in patients with skin cancer. British Journal of Dermatology, 185(3):654–655, 2021.

91. Ishan Asokan, Soniya V Rabadia, and Eric H Yang. The COVID-19 pandemic and its impact on the cardio-oncology population. Current Oncology Reports, 22:1–13, 2020.

92. Yifan Meng, Wanrong Lu, Ensong Guo, et al. Cancer history is an independent risk factor for mortality in hospitalized COVID-19 patients: A propensity score-matched analysis. Journal of Hematology & Oncology, 13(1):1–11, 2020.

93. TW Andrew, M Alrawi, and P Lovat. Reduction in skin cancer diagnoses in the UK during the COVID-19 pandemic. Clinical and Experimental Dermatology, 46(1):145–146, 2021.

94. Luca Tagliaferri, Alessandro Di Stefani, Giovanni Schinzari, et al. Skin cancer triage and management during COVID-19 pandemic. Journal of the European Academy of Dermatology and Venereology, 34(6):1136–1139, 2020.

95. N Howlader, AM Noone, M Krapcho, et al. Seer cancer statistics review, 1975–2018. National Cancer Institute, pp. 1–25, 2021.

96. Australian Institute of Health and Welfare. The first year of COVID-19 in Australia: Direct and indirect health effects. www.aihw.gov.au/reports/burden-of-disease/the-first-year-of-COVID-19-in-australia/summary, 2021. Accessed 8 December 2021.

97. Australian Government Department of Health. Palliative care. www.health.gov.au/health-topics/palliative-care?utm source=health.gov.au&utm medium=redirect&utm campaign=digital transformation&utm content=pa 2021. Accessed 14 October 2021.

98. Steven P Cohen, Zafeer B Baber, Asokumar Buvanendran, et al. Pain management best practices from multispecialty organizations during the COVID-19 pandemic and public health crises. Pain Medicine, 21(7):1331–1346, 2020.

99. Marco A Cimmino, Carmela Ferrone, and Maurizio Cutolo. Epidemiology of chronic musculoskeletal pain. Best Practice & Research Clinical Rheumatology, 25(2):173–183, 2011.

100. The Lancet. Palliative care and the COVID-19 pandemic. Lancet (London, England), 395(10231):1168, 2020.

101. Xue Jun Song, Dong Lin Xiong, Zhe Yin Wang, et al. Pain management during the COVID-19 pandemic in China: Lessons learned. Pain Medicine, 21(7):1319–1323, 2020.

102. Filomena Puntillo, Mariateresa Giglio, Nicola Brienza, et al. Impact of COVID-19 pandemic on chronic pain management: Looking for the best way to deliver care. Best Practice & Research Clinical Anaesthesiology, 34(3):529–537, 2020.

103. Simon N Etkind, Anna E Bone, Natasha Lovell, et al. The role and response of palliative care and hospice services in epidemics and pandemics: A rapid review to inform practice during the COVID-19 pandemic. Journal of Pain and Symptom Management, 60(1):e31-e40, 2020.

104. Jane DeLima Thomas, Richard E Leiter, Janet L Abrahm, et al. Development of a palliative care toolkit for the COVID-19 pandemic. Journal of Pain and Symptom Management, 60(2):e22-e25, 2020.

105. Lukas Radbruch, Felicia Marie Knaul, Liliana de Lima, et al. The key role of palliative care in response to the COVID-19 tsunami of suffering. The Lancet, 395(10235):1467–1469, 2020.

106. Felicia Marie Knaul, Paul E Farmer, Eric L Krakauer, et al. Alleviating the access abyss in palliative care and pain relief—An imperative of universal health coverage: The Lancet Commission report. The Lancet, 391(10128):1391–1454, 2018.

107. Amit Arya, Sandy Buchman, Bruno Gagnon, and James Downar. Pandemic palliative care: Beyond ventilators and saving lives. Canadian Medical Association Journal, 192(15):E400-E404, 2020.

108. Victoria D Powell and Maria J Silveira. What should palliative care's response be to the COVID-19 pandemic? Journal of Pain and Symptom Management, 60(1):e1-e3, 2020.

109. Laura C Hanson, Barbara Usher, Lynn Spragens, and Stephen Bernard. Clinical and economic impact of palliative care consultation. Journal of Pain and Symptom Management, 35(4):340–346, 2008.

110. Pradeep Rangappa, Karthik Rao, Thrilok Chandra, et al. Tele-medicine, telerounds, and tele-intensive care unit in the COVID-19 pandemic. Indian Journal of Medical Specialties, 12(1):4, 2021.

111. Aaron K Wong, Lucy Demediuk, Jia Y Tay, et al. COVID-19 end-of-life care: Symptoms and supportive therapy use in an Australian hospital. Internal Medicine Journal, 51(9):1420–1425, 2021.

112. Natasha Lovell, Matthew Maddocks, Simon N Etkind, et al. Characteristics, symptom management, and outcomes of 101 patients with COVID-19 referred for hospital palliative care. Journal of Pain and Symptom Management, 60(1):e77-e81, 2020.

113. Emma Hack, Barbara Hayes, Nicholas Radcliffe, et al. COVID-19 pandemic: End of life experience in Australian residential aged care facilities. Internal Medicine Journal, 10–111, 2021.

114. Jennifer Currin-McCulloch, Brooke Chapman, Colleen Carson, et al. Hearts above water: Palliative care during a pandemic. Social Work in Health Care, 60(1):93–105, 2021.

115. Advance Care Planning Australia. Advance care planning and COVID-19. www.advancecareplanning.org.au/understand-advance-care-planning/advance-care-planning-and-covid-19, 2021. Accessed 20 February 2022.

116. Andy Bradshaw, Lesley Dunleavy, Catherine Walshe, et al. Understanding and addressing challenges for advance care planning in the COVID-19 pandemic: An analysis of the UK CovPall survey data from specialist palliative care services. Palliative Medicine, 35(7):1225–1237, 2021.

117. Salah N El-Tallawy, Rohit Nalamasu, Joseph V Pergolizzi, and Christopher Gharibo. Pain management during the COVID-19 pandemic. Pain and Therapy, 9(2):453–466, 2020.

118. Palliative Care Australia. Palliative Care Australia Strategic Direction 2022–2024. https://palliativecare.org.au/publication/palliative-care-australia-strategic-direction-2022–2024/, 2022. Accessed 22 February 2022.

119. Australian Government Department of Health. Medicare benefits schedule book category 6 operating from 1 March 2021. www.mbsonline.gov.au/internet/mbsonline/publishing.nsf/Content/4EFCF78281A91736CA2586540011 38AF/File/202103-cat6.pdf, 2021. Accessed 10 November 2021.

CHAPTER 3

Estimating the Relative Contribution of Transmission to the Prevalence of Drug Resistance in Tuberculosis

Tanzila K. Chowdhury, Laurence A.F. Park, Glenn Stone, Mark M Tanaka, and Andrew Francis

3.1 INTRODUCTION

Tuberculosis (TB) is a respiratory infectious disease caused by the bacterium *Mycobacterium tuberculosis*. The World Health Organization (WHO) estimates that about 1.5 million people died in 2020 due to tuberculosis [2020]. The TB latent and infectious period span long time intervals (years on average) and reduce rapidly two weeks after effective treatment is initiated [Ozcaglar et al., 2012]. The most common first-line drugs used to treat TB are rifampicin, isoniazid, ethambutol, streptomycin, and pyrazinamide, but the acquisition of resistance to these drugs has been a growing problem [Diriba et al., 2013]. Indeed, multi–drug-resistant tuberculosis (MDR TB), defined as resistance to isoniazid (INH) and rifampicin (RIF), is an increasing global problem [Espinal, 2003]. There are even some cases of "extensive" drug resistance (XDR), defined as MDR cases

DOI: 10.1201/9781003292357-3

with additional resistance to fluoroquinolone and at least one second-line injectable agent (kanamycin, amikacin, or capreomycin) [Diriba et al., 2013]. Once tuberculosis becomes extensively resistant, it requires very expensive and extensive treatment [Wright et al., 2006]. Compounding the challenge, less affluent countries bear the highest burden of TB, and people with HIV are more likely to develop active TB. In 2020, the 30 highest TB-burdened countries accounted for 86% of new TB cases. Eight countries account for two-thirds of the total, with India leading the count, followed by China, Indonesia, the Philippines, Pakistan, Nigeria, Bangladesh, and South Africa [WHO, 2020].

Understanding the mechanisms and patterns of resistance evolution is both urgent and essential to controlling TB spread. There are two possible ways for a patient to have acquired drug-resistant tuberculosis. The first is through acquiring resistance while infected (resistance evolution or treatment failure), and the second is by transmission (infection with an already-resistant strain). We are interested to know how the state of being drug sensitive or drug resistant is reached. For example, if we observe five resistant cases in an outbreak sample, these resistant cases either occurred via transmission or treatment failure. It is possible that only one person acquired the resistance because they did not administer their treatment properly (treatment failure) and then transmitted a resistant strain to four other people. This is only one of the five possibilities, and another extreme possibility is that all cases of resistance were acquired independently. If public health authorities know which way of acquiring infection with a resistant strain (transmission or treatment failure) is more common, the public health system can use this to take the necessary steps to stop the spread of resistant TB. That is, if we find that resistance was mostly acquired through treatment failure, the health system needs to ensure that effective treatment procedures are in place. On the other hand, if resistance was acquired mainly due to transmission, there needs to be a more robust system in place to control TB transmission.

The purpose of this chapter is to describe an efficient method to estimate the relative contributions of transmission, and treatment failure, to the spread of drug resistance in an outbreak. Luciani et al. [2009] estimated the relative contribution of transmission to the spread of TB drug resistance using approximate Bayesian computation (ABC) and a transmission-mutation model, which produced posterior distributions of key parameters of interest. More recent studies, such as Rodrigues et al. [2018], have also used ABC to look at the relative contribution problem in the context of multiple drug resistance. However, the process of ABC is computationally heavy and hence time-consuming, taking days to provide a result and longer to fine-tune the model. In this chapter, we investigate a simple method for approximating the parameters of a TB outbreak that produces results in minutes. We also evaluate the accuracy of the computed parameters under different conditions. The contribution of our research is a simpler model that produces quick estimation and predicts similar results to the Luciani et al. [2009] analysis. No other studies are known that efficiently estimate the relative contribution of transmission and evolution in the spread of TB drug resistance. The two main advantages of the method described in this chapter are its efficiency and simplicity of calculation, relative to a method such as ABC. If a healthcare worker wants to understand the TB transmission mechanism to decide on the steps/treatment to control TB resistance, getting a quick result will be an advantage over the time and expertise required to get results using an ABC approach. Additionally, people with minimal programming knowledge can use the method we describe; it does not need field experts to estimate the relative contributions to TB transmission.

We will use data from several published sources: Bolivia [Monteserin et al., 2013], Tanzania [Kibiki et al., 2007], Cuba [Diaz et al., 1998], and Chad [Diguimbaye et al., 2006]. These sources provide essential tuberculosis genotypic information and drug resistance information for several first-line drugs: isoniazid, rifampicin, pyrazinamide, streptomycin, and ethambutol. Each dataset has several clusters of isolates and information about their phenotype (drug resistance).

The layout of the chapter is as follows. Section 3.2 describes the structure and the visualisation of the data according to their genotype and drug resistance information. We will define a *resistance acquisition graph* for a single cluster and the most probable event history of that cluster in Sections 3.3 and 3.4. Once we have the resistance acquisition graph of a cluster, we can extend this process to a set of clusters, as explained in Section 3.5. This allows us to achieve the chapter's key goal, to make estimates of the proportion of drug resistance cases that have arisen from the transmission. We have included some analysis of our method in Section 3.6.

3.2 SPOLIGOFORESTS WITH DRUG-RESISTANCE INFORMATION

3.2.1 Spoligoforests

While several genotyping methods can be used to characterise variation in bacterial pathogens, this study is based on a technique known as spacer oligonucleotide typing or spoligotyping. Spoligotyping is a rapid poly-merase chain reaction (PCR)-based method for genotyping strains of the TB complex [Kamerbeek et al., 1997], developed to provide information on the structure of the direct repeat (DR) region in individual TB strains and different members of the TB complex [Streicher et al., 2007]. This method determines the presence or absence of 43 different spacers. The binary string representing the pattern of the presence or absence of spacers in a given isolate constitutes a spoligotype. The data used for this research are based on tuberculosis isolates typed with spoligotyping (see Figure 3.2) and phenotypic information relating to antibacterial drug resistance. While more sophisticated genotyping techniques such as whole genome sequencing (WGS) are now available, spoligotyping remains widely used in public health and epidemiological contexts, because it is cheap, fast, and reliable, and in many countries the cost of WGS means it is not widely available.

Given a dataset of spoligotyped isolates, we can form clusters of isolates with identical spoligotypes and then construct *spoligoforests* with directed edges between clusters [Reyes et al., 2008]. Spoligotyping information is used to construct a spoligoforest of the outbreak sample. Inside a spoligo-forest, an arrow goes from cluster A to cluster B if A is the parent of B; that is, the genotype of cluster B evolved from that of cluster A. Assuming there is no homoplasy (when a trait has been gained or lost independently over the course of evolution), a spoligotype can only arise from a single parent spoligotype. However, multiple child clusters can appear from a single par-ent cluster. A sample spoligoforest is shown in Figure 3.1.

Aside from the genotype, which here is defined by spoligotyping, each cluster in the spoligoforest may have both drug-sensitive and drug-resistant

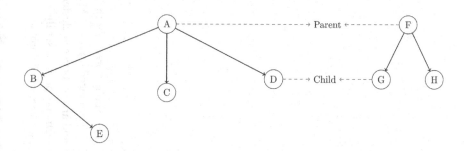

FIGURE 3.1   A sample spoligoforest. Here, A is the parent cluster of B, C, and D clusters, and F is the parent of G and H. B is the parent of child cluster E. Genotype of a child cluster is a genetic evolution from the parent cluster.

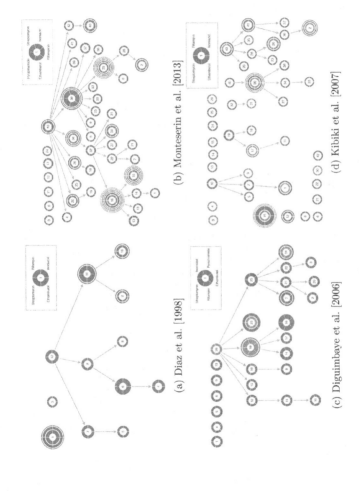

FIGURE 3.2 Spoligoforests for the datasets taken from Diaz et al. [1998], Monteserin et al. [2013], Diguimbaye et al. [2006], and Kibiki et al. [2007] produced using the MERCAT package [Aandahl et al., 2020]. Each disc represents a cluster of isolates with the same spoligotype, and arrows between clusters represent likely single-step spoligotype mutations. The area of each disc represents the size of the cluster, segments of the discs illustrate drug resistance states for drugs as shown in each legend, and concentric bands indicate isolates with the same resistance profile.

isolates. That is, the cluster is defined by a single genotype but may contain more than one phenotype.

3.2.2 Visualising Spoligoforests with Drug Resistance Information

For a given set of isolates typed with spoligotyping, one can construct a spoligoforest following the methods of Reyes et al. [2008]. This represents a possible mutational history, showing single step directional edges and resolving potential homoplasy to choose a single parent for each cluster (using the method of Ozcaglar et al. [2012]).

While in this study we focus on the simple phenotypes of "sensitive" or "resistant" in relation to a given drug, the methods in MERCAT [Aandahl et al., 2020] allow the visual representation of a range of possible drug resistance "profiles" for each cluster of isolates with identical spoligotype. We have used spoligotyping and phenotypic (drug resistance) information from published datasets. Using this information, MERCAT can construct spoligoforests for the sample. Figure 3.2 shows such spoligoforests of four different datasets labelled accordingly: Diaz et al. [1998] (12 clusters), Monteserin et al. [2013] (43 clusters), Diguimbaye et al. [2006] (26 clusters), and Kibiki et al. [2007] (43 clusters). These graphs were produced using MERCAT [Aandahl et al., 2020]. A summary of all four datasets showing resistance information is given in Table 3.1. These datasets have drug resistance information for five different drugs, rifampicin (RIF), isoniazid (INH), ethambutol (EMB), streptomycin (STR), and pyrazinamide (PZA).

Each node in the spoligoforest produced by MERCAT denotes a genotype cluster. Each concentric band indicates isolates in the cluster with the same drug resistance "profile", and the area of the band is proportional to the number of isolates with that profile (an isolate carrying a drug resistance "profile" means it is resistant to a subset of drugs and sensitive to the remaining drugs). The resistance status of isolates in the cluster with respect to any given drug is then represented in a "pizza slice". The green label indicates sensitivity, the orange label indicates resistance, and the blue label indicates "not identified" cases.

3.3 THE RESISTANCE ACQUISITION GRAPH FOR A SINGLE CLUSTER

This section describes our approach for a single cluster of isolates with identical genotypes. We summarise each cluster with two numbers: drug-sensitive cases (i) and drug-resistant cases (j) as an ordered pair (i, j).

TABLE 3.1   Numbers of Resistant Isolates in the Datasets from Diaz et al. [1998], Monteserin et al. [2013], Diguimbaye et al. [2006], and Kibiki et al. [2007]. We have information for five different drugs collected from these datasets: rifampicin (RIF), isoniazid (INH), ethambutol (EMB), streptomycin (STR), and pyrazinamide (PZA). Pan-sensitive refers to sensitivity to all drugs. Note that some isolates carry resistance to more than one drug.

Drug	Diaz	Monteserin	Diguimbaye	Kibiki
RIF	3	6	0	3
INH	1	8	9	11
EMB	0	7	4	3
STR	16	4	0	4
PZA	—	1	3	—
Pan-sensitive	58	21	19	98
Total isolates	74	35	32	110

For instance, a cluster with one sensitive case and two resistant cases is denoted by (1, 2). Each cluster has several possible histories, beginning with a single source case. We represent these possible historical paths by a *resistance acquisition graph*, which is a directed graph whose vertices represent the state of clusters of one strain. This figure shows all the possible paths by which the cluster may have arisen from a single source case under the assumption that all cases are observed.

We will establish several rules to calculate the "most probable events" (MPEs) on the graph for different clusters. Using this approach, we will determine the most probable evolutionary events of different cluster phenotypes and calculate the frequencies of various evolutionary events (transmission and treatment failure). In the next section, we will combine information from each component cluster in the spoligoforest.

The directed edges in the graph indicate two types of events: the acquisition of drug resistance and the transmission of the pathogen. Edges marking a treatment failure event are labelled A (for acquisition) and indicate the movement of an isolate from sensitive status to resistant status: $(i, j) \rightarrow (i - 1, j + 1)$. Such edges are only possible if the cluster has sensitive cases: if $i \geq 1$. Edges marking a resistance transmission event indicate either transmission of a sensitive case $((i, j) \rightarrow (i + 1, j))$ or a resistant case $((i, j) \rightarrow (i, j + 1))$ and are labelled T_s and T_r, respectively. The edges described previously allow only three types of vertices (cluster). These vertex types are: all sensitive $(i, 0)$, all resistant $(0, j)$, or mixed (i, j). The possible edges for each of these types are shown in Figure 3.3.

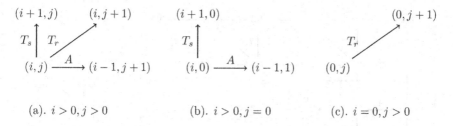

(a). $i > 0, j > 0$ (b). $i > 0, j = 0$ (c). $i = 0, j > 0$

FIGURE 3.3   General rules for all possible events of three different types of clusters. Here, (a) represents a cluster with both sensitive and resistant cases, (b) represents clusters consisting of sensitive cases only, and (c) represents clusters with resistant cases only. All types of events (T_s, T_r, and A) are possible for (a), whereas only T_s and A are possible for (b), and only T_r is possible for (c).

Note that in this model, we assume that the source of a cluster is a single isolate, in accordance with the infinite alleles model (no homoplasy) [Reyes et al., 2012]. We also assume that resistance, once gained, is not lost (following Luciani et al. [2009]). This means that a cluster with sensitive cases *must* have a sensitive case as the source.

As an example, the resistance acquisition graph for the cluster (1, 2) is shown in Figure 3.4 (right). Three possible paths can lead a single sensitive case (1, 0) to a final position (1, 2). Depending on which path we take, the number of transmission and evolution events are different. Two of these paths include two sensitive transmissions (T_s) and two resistance evolution (A) events. Another path includes one sensitive transmission (T_s), one resistant transmission (T_r), and one resistance evolution (A) event. The resistance acquisition graph for a cluster (0, 5) is shown in Figure 3.4.

Each cluster is associated with its own resistance acquisition graph within the spoligoforest. Once we can calculate the relative contribution of resistance transmission and treatment failure in a cluster, we can extend that approach to all possible clusters in the spoligoforest. This way, we will be able to calculate the proportion of resistance due to transmission/ treatment failure for the whole sample and then for the entire outbreak by accounting for the weighting factor. Figure 3.5 shows a sample spoligoforest and the approach to studying various events within an outbreak. In Section 3.5, we will discuss how to combine information across clusters in the spoligoforest to study the whole outbreak.

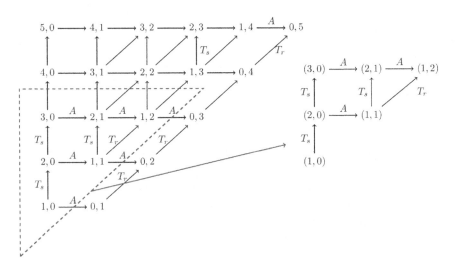

FIGURE 3.4 The resistance acquisition graph for a cluster with five resistant strains (0, 5) is shown on the left. We omit parentheses for simplicity. Note that *all* resistance acquisition graphs for clusters of sizes up to 5 are included in this figure. The graph for a cluster with one sensitive strain and two resistant strains (1, 2) is shown on the right. Here, (1, 0) is the source (bottom left), and (1, 2) is the final position of this cluster (top right corner). Arrows inside the graph indicate the evolution of drug resistance (labelled *A*) or the transmission of sensitive or resistant strains (T_s and T_r, respectively).

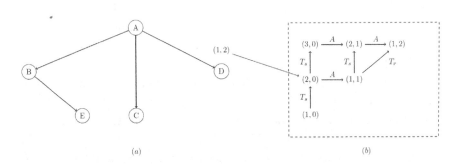

FIGURE 3.5 A sample spoligoforest (a). Within this spoligoforest, we can construct a resistance acquisition graph for each cluster. An example of the resistance acquisition graph of cluster D is shown here (b). This cluster has one sensitive case and two resistant cases.

3.4 HISTORY OF A CLUSTER

In the previous section, we saw that several possible paths through the resistance acquisition graph lead to the final observed cluster. While each path in the graph may correspond to many parallel sequences of events (for instance, the edge $(2, 0) \rightarrow (1, 1)$ could correspond to the acquisition of drug resistance by either of the two isolates in the initial cluster), in this section, we consider which *individual* path is the most probable.

The probability of each path through the resistance acquisition graph is proportional to the product of the probabilities of the events that occurred on each step of that path. Let α, τ_s, τ_r be the rates of evolution/treatment failure, sensitive transmission, and resistant transmission per individual per unit time (year), respectively. The probability of a particular path to the cluster (i, j) is determined by the frequencies of the different events along the path. For instance, the path $(1, 0) \rightarrow (2, 0) \rightarrow (1, 1) \rightarrow (1, 2)$ in Figure 3.4 has one sensitive transmission, one resistant transmission, and one evolution of drug resistance event, so the probability of the path is given by the product $\tau_s \tau_r 2\alpha$. The number 2 before α is included because this represents the edge probability of $(2, 0) \rightarrow (1, 1)$, and there are two sensitive cases in that edge, both of which can acquire resistance. However, the path $(1, 0) \rightarrow (2, 0) \rightarrow (1, 1) \rightarrow (2, 1) \rightarrow (1, 2)$ in Figure 3.4 has two sensitive transmissions and two evolutions of drug resistance, so the probability of the path is given by the product $\tau^2 (2 \times 2) \, \alpha^2$. Therefore, we need to consider the frequency of the events in the path as well as, sometimes, the multiplicities of sensitive or resistant cases in each position of the path. If we can compute the probability of every path in the resistance acquisition graph, we can determine the most probable history of an observed cluster.

However, this requires calculating probabilities of each edge, and the number of edges increases rapidly as the cluster sizes increase. As an alternative, we will look at the most probable events along the path, which ignores the frequency of different cases at each position along the path. This method produces results efficiently and provides an easily computable proxy for the most probable path of an observed cluster. In future work, we will compare this proxy with a more complete study of the most probable path through the resistance acquisition graph, but for the present, we will assess this proxy against known parameters in simulations (Section 6).

For the specific example shown in Figure 3.4 (right), there are three paths from $(1, 0)$ to $(1, 2)$, and each path has probability proportional to either $\tau^2\alpha^2$ or $\tau_s\alpha\tau_r$. We summarise these frequencies in a vector of three integers so that we represent the probability $\tau^a\tau^b\alpha^c$ by the triple (a, b, c) of exponents, where a, b, and c are the frequency of sensitive transmission, resistant transmission, and treatment failure events, respectively. The most probable events for a cluster (i, j) will correspond to a particular triple of exponents, which we denote $\varepsilon_{(i,j)}$. This triple depends on whether the root of the cluster is a sensitive or resistant case $((1, 0)$ or $(0, 1))$, so we will often make this clear with a superscript, $\varepsilon_{(i,j)}^{(1,0)}$ or $\varepsilon_{(i,j)}^{(0,1)}$.

The main result of this section is the following proposition, which gives the most probable event history to any cluster from a sensitive source case.

Proposition 1. *The most probable events history of the cluster (i, j) from source $(1, 0)$ with different rates $\tau_s = 0.66$, $\tau_r = 0.60$, and $\alpha = 0.01$ has event frequencies for T_s, T_r, and A events given as follows:*

$$\varepsilon_{(i,j)}^{(1,0)} = \begin{cases} (i, j-1, 1) & \text{if } i \geq 0, j > 0, \text{ and} \\ (i-1, 0, 0) & \text{if } i > 0, j = 0 \end{cases} \tag{1}$$

Proof. In the resistance acquisition graph (see Figure 3.4), the (i, j) cluster is j steps to the right and $i + j - 1$ steps above the source isolate $(1, 0)$. There are two types of steps to move above: sensitive transmissions (T_s) and resistant transmissions (T_r), and two types of steps to move right: resistant transmission (T_r) and resistance evolution (A) events. Suppose that on a given path π, there are (a) sensitive transmissions (T_s), (b) resistant transmissions (T_r), and (c) resistance evolution (A) events. Then this implies $a + b = i + j - 1$ (the number of steps up), and $b + c = j$ (the number of steps to the right). Making b the object, we have

$$a = \cdot i + j - 1 \cdot - b$$

$$c = \cdot j - b$$

Note that b is between 0 and j but is strictly less than j since an initial resistance evolution must occur so that $0 \leq b \leq j - 1$ and hence $c > 0$. We can calculate the value, which is proportional to the probability of this path, $P(\pi)$, as follows.

$$P(\pi) = \alpha^{j-b}\tau_s^{i+j-1-b}\tau_r^b = \alpha^j\tau_s^{i+j-1}\left(\frac{\tau_r}{\alpha\tau_s}\right)^b \tag{2}$$

Since i and j are fixed by the cluster, maximising this probability reduces to choosing a path with the maximal number of resistant transmissions (b), as long as the ratio $\dfrac{Tr}{\alpha Ts}$ is more than 1.

Previous studies showed that, in general, the rate at which resistant transmissions occur is significantly higher than the rate of resistance acquisition events, or $\tau_r > \alpha$ [Luciani et al., 2009]. That paper estimated the rates of sensitive transmission, resistant transmission, and resistance acquisition to be 0.66, 0.6, and 0.01, which forces $\dfrac{Tr}{\alpha Ts}$ to be more than 1.

Assuming $j > 0$, the highest possible value of b is $j - 1$, and choosing this value forces $a = i$ and $c = 1$, as required by the statement of the proposition. On the other hand, when $j = 0$, the relation $c = j - b$ forces c to be negative unless $b = 0$. Consequently, $b = c = 0$, and $a = i + j - 1 - b = i - 1$, giving $\varepsilon_{(i,j)}^{(1,0)} = (i - 1, 0, 0)$, as required by the proposition.

In some of what follows, we will consider the situation in which there is a single resistant case as the source for a cluster (such a cluster necessarily only consists of resistant isolates). In that case, there will be one less acquisition of drug resistance than with a sensitive case as a source: we remove the step $(1, 0) \rightarrow (0, 1)$. This argument gives the following lemma:

Lemma 4.2. *When the source is a single resistant case $(0, 1)$ for a cluster of resistant strains $(0, j)$, there will be one less drug resistance acquisition than with the sensitive source. In this case, for $i = 0, j > 0$,*
$$\varepsilon_{(i,j)}^{(1,0)} = (0, j - 1, 0).$$

3.5 BEYOND A SINGLE CLUSTER

In this section, we will extend our method of calculating the transmission proportion for a single cluster to the whole outbreak. Moving from the single-cluster analysis given in the previous sections to evaluating a multi-cluster outbreak requires summing over the clusters and accounting for connections between clusters in the spoligoforest. This section shows how to do this, beginning with the issues around choosing a source for each cluster. Appointing a source for a cluster is essential, as we need to account for the event that has happened to start a new cluster. If the source of an observed cluster is $(1, 0)$, a sensitive transmission happens from the ancestor cluster to the source of the observed cluster. However, if the source of an observed cluster is the resistant case $(0, 1)$, then a resistance acquisition event occurred from the ancestor cluster to the source of the observed cluster. This is explained in detail in section 3.5.2.

3.5.1 Assigning the Source Isolate

In studying a single cluster, we accounted for two alternatives for the source isolate: it could be either drug sensitive $(1, 0)$ or drug resistant $(0, 1)$. In what follows, we will describe how this choice of source can be forced by the wider context of the cluster or chosen based on the parsimonious approach used in this research.

We have assumed that resistance cannot be lost for an individual isolate. This has an effect on the source of a cluster in some situations: if the cluster has any drug-sensitive cases, then the source of the cluster must have been sensitive. On the other hand, if the cluster contains only resistant cases, then the assumption that resistance cannot be lost does not rule out either possible source. However, that assumption can still have an impact on the source of the cluster, depending on the descendants of the cluster.

Specifically, if we know that one of the descendants of an all resistant cluster has a sensitive root source, then since the descendant cluster's genotype evolved from the ancestor cluster's genotype, this source case was originally a member of the ancestor cluster. This forces the source of the ancestor cluster to have been a sensitive case. In other words: a sensitive source in the descendant forces a sensitive source in the ancestor.

If none of the descendant clusters of an all resistant cluster has sensitive sources, then we need to look at the ancestor cluster. If the ancestor cluster has no resistant cases, then somewhere in between the clusters, the acquisition of drug resistance occurred. Therefore, for simplicity, we will assume that the source of these types of clusters ($(0, j)$ cluster with $(0, j)$ descendant and $(i, 0)$ ancestor) is a sensitive source.

Finally, suppose our cluster has no sensitive case, none of its descendant clusters has a sensitive source, and the ancestor cluster consists of resistant cases ($(0, j)$ cluster with $(0, j)$ descendant and (i, j) or $(0, j)$ ancestor); then the most probable event path is from a source that is a single resistant case.

To summarise, the rules we follow to assign a source to a cluster (i, j) are described in Proposition 2.

Proposition 2. *Assuming that resistance once attained, cannot be lost and that there is no homoplasy, the source of a cluster (i, j) that has arisen from the most probable event path from a single isolate is given in the following cases:*

(1) *Cluster (i, j) or $(i, 0)$: If there are sensitive cases in a cluster $(i > 0)$, the source is a sensitive case $(1, 0)$.*

(2) *Cluster $(0, j)$: If there is no sensitive case in a cluster $(i = 0)$, the source is dependent on the ancestor and descendant clusters, as follows:*

    (a) *Descendant cluster (i, j) or $(i, 0)$: If there is a descendant cluster with sensitive cases $(i > 0)$, the source of the cluster $(0, j)$ is a sensitive case $(1, 0)$.*

    (b) *Descendant cluster $(0, j)$: If the descendant cluster consists of resistant cases only:*

        (i) *Ancestor cluster $(i, 0)$: If the ancestor cluster consists of sensitive cases only, the source of the cluster $(0, j)$ is a sensitive case $(1, 0)$.*

        (ii) *Ancestor cluster (i, j) or $(0, j)$: If the ancestor cluster consists of resistant cases, the source is a resistant case $(0, 1)$.*

This proposition gives an algorithm for assigning drug resistance status to source isolates of clusters in a spoligoforest. We first determine the source of clusters that have no descendants. Their ancestors can then have their sources determined, and so on. The decision behind the allocation of sources moves from the descendant to the ancestor.

3.5.2 Event Calculations for the Whole Sample

This section describes how to compute the totals of different events (sensitive and resistant transmission and treatment failure) across the whole sample. The next step is summing the totals of each event from each cluster once sources have been assigned according to the previous section. However, we must also account for events that give rise to the source case, which may involve looking at the ancestor of each cluster.

The source case of a cluster is the first with its particular genotype. This evolution of genotype is assumed to occur independently of resistance evolution and transmission dynamics. Therefore, the source case acquired its resistance status from an event, and this is what we need to count.

If the source case is *sensitive*, then it must have arisen from a sensitive transmission T_s. This transmission would have occurred within the ancestor cluster before the genotype evolution but is not counted there: we will count it in the cluster where the source case occurs.

We have denoted the count of events for the most probable event path in the cluster with a sensitive source by the triplet $\varepsilon_{(i,j)}^{(1,0)} = (a, b, c)$, where a, b, and c are the number of sensitive transmission, resistant transmission, and treatment failure events, respectively. We will denote the augmented count by $\varepsilon^{\circ}{}_{(i,j)}^{(1,0)}$ which includes the event for the source isolate. The previous discussion shows:

$$\varepsilon^{\circ}{}_{(i,j)}^{(1,0)} = \varepsilon_{(i,j)}^{(1,0)} + (1,0,0)$$

Suppose the source isolate is drug *resistant*. In that case, there are two possible ways it could have arisen from a resistant transmission T_r (from another resistant isolate) or resistance evolution A (from a sensitive isolate). To select which of these to count, we need to inspect the ancestor cluster.

For a cluster to have a resistant source, there are two cases for the ancestor cluster: it could consist entirely of resistant cases $(0, j)$ or of a mixture of both (i, j) (Proposition 1). If the ancestor cluster consists of entirely drug-resistant cases, it must have arisen from a resistant transmission. If the ancestor cluster contains both sensitive and resistant cases, then the source case of the descendant may have arisen from either a drug-resistant transmission or an evolution. However, considering both clusters as a single system, the most probable event path would have a single drug evolution, and this would already be counted in the ancestor cluster. So we take the source isolate to have arisen from a resistant transmission.

In other words, $\varepsilon^{\circ}{}_{(i,j)}^{(1,0)} = \varepsilon_{(i,j)}^{(1,0)} + (1,0,0)$ if the ancestor cluster is all resistant or mixed.

In summary, we have

$$\varepsilon^{\circ}{}_{(i,j)}^{(1,0)} = \begin{cases} (i,0,0 \\ (i+1, j-1, 1 \end{cases} \quad \text{if the cluster is all sensitive and otherwise.}$$

$$\varepsilon^{\circ}{}_{(i,j)}^{(1,0)} = \varepsilon_{(i,j)}^{(1,0)} + (1,0,0) \quad \text{for all cases}$$

Note that we have assigned a sensitive source for a root cluster of the spoligoforest, which has no ancestor clusters. In this case, there is not enough information about the origin of the source case, and for simplicity, we assume that the source is a sensitive case $(1, 0)$.

The inference described here is deterministic, allowing us to infer the numbers of events directly from cluster structure. In particular, the

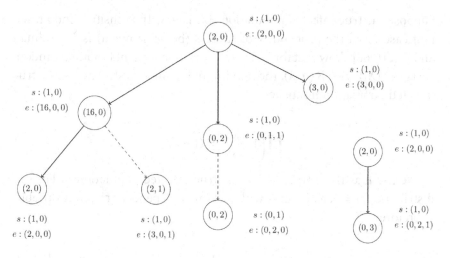

FIGURE 3.6 Spoligoforest for data from Monteserin et al. [2013], focusing on resistance to isoniazid. This graph corresponds to the second row of the Monteserin column in Table 3.1. Each circle represents a cluster with (i, j), meaning i sensitive and j resistant cases. The source of each cluster (s: $(1, 0)/(0, 1)$) and the frequency of events ($e = (T_s, T_r, A)$) are shown next to each cluster.

numbers of resistant and sensitive cases in an isolated cluster determine the proportion of resistant cases due to transmission. In the generic case of a cluster with i sensitive and j resistant cases ($i, j > 0$), the proportion of resistant cases due to transmission is inferred to be $\dfrac{b}{b+c} = \dfrac{j-1}{j}$ (Proposition 1).

An example of assigning sources to clusters, as described in Proposition 2, is shown in Figure 3.6. This figure accommodates all the rules we have introduced to calculate different events for the whole spoligoforest.

3.5.3 Accounting for Sampling

The data we observe represent only a sample of an underlying infected outbreak. To estimate the parameters of an infected outbreak, the next step is to account for sampling weights so that our sample represents the infected outbreak. We assume that the process of sampling follows a binomial distribution with two outcomes: success indicates we have successfully sampled the case from an outbreak (we observe this in the sample), and failure indicates that we have failed to sample the case from an outbreak. We assume that sampling is not biased with respect to resistance and that there is an equal chance of sampling a sensitive or resistant case.

Suppose the true infected population size is n, with i sensitive and j resistant cases, and the probability of success (being sampled) is λ. Feldman and Fox [1968] show that for k ($k = 1, \ldots, r$) independent binomial random variables (X_k) with $B(n, \lambda)$, the maximum likelihood estimate for the true infected population n satisfies:

$$\prod_{k=1}^{r}\left(1 - \frac{x_k}{\hat{n}}\right) = (1 - \lambda)^r \tag{3}$$

We use $\hat{n}$ as the estimation of the true infected population n. For our distribution, $r = 1$, as we deal with just one independent random variable. Therefore:

$$1 - \frac{x}{\hat{n}} = 1 - \lambda$$

$$\hat{n} = \frac{x}{\lambda} \tag{4}$$

Therefore, we can scale up the observed cluster (i, j) by dividing the sampling proportion. That is, for sampling proportion $\lambda \in (0, 1]$, we scale up each cluster so that (i, j) becomes $\left(\dfrac{i}{\lambda}, \dfrac{j}{\lambda}\right)$ In particular, if a cluster has zero sensitive or resistant cases, this stays zero. As we are dealing with TB cases, we have rounded the result for simplicity.

3.5.4 The Effect of Sampling on the Proportion of Resistance due to Transmission

To calculate the proportion of resistance due to transmission for an outbreak, we need to consider the sampling behind the data. Keeping the proportions of sensitive and resistant cases constant in a cluster, as the cluster size grows, the inferred proportion of resistance due to transmission also grows.

Suppose the true cluster size is m, with j resistant cases. If the sampling proportion is λ, then the cluster size of the sample is λm with λj resistant cases. The inferred proportion of resistant cases arising from transmission will be $\dfrac{\lambda j - 1}{\lambda j} = 1 - \dfrac{1}{\lambda j}$, while the true proportion should be $\dfrac{j-1}{j} = 1 - \dfrac{1}{j}$. Since $\lambda j \cdot <= \cdot j$, the effect of sampling is to underestimate the proportion of resistant cases due to transmission.

However, we can make a simple correction if we know the sampling proportion or estimate it from the TB yearly reports prepared by WHO. If we have sampled j^t and the estimated sampling proportion is λ, then our estimate of the infected population level proportion of drug resistance due to transmission is $\dfrac{(j/\lambda)-1}{j/\lambda} = \dfrac{j-\lambda}{j}$. That is, instead of a proportion of $\dfrac{j-1}{j}$, we use $\dfrac{j-\lambda}{j}$. which is just $1-\dfrac{1}{j}$ since $j^t = \lambda j$.

3.6 RESULTS

3.6.1 Results, Comparison with Simulation

Once we have the MPE model ready, the next logical step is to test the model to check whether it predicts an accurate measure. In this section, we show the results of the method using a simulation study. To do this, we will compare the result of our model with simulated outbreaks. We will simulate hundreds of outbreaks to predict the parameters of interest (resistance due to transmission and treatment failure). In the simulation process, we know exactly how many different types of events (T_r or A) occur throughout the process. We will compare these numbers with the result from the MPE model.

We initialise the simulation from a single sensitive case $(1, 0)$. For any position (i, j) in the simulation, five possible edges indicate five possible events: sensitive transmission, resistant transmission, resistance evolution (treatment failure), sensitive death or recovery, and resistant death or recovery. Using the parameter values estimated by Luciani et al. [2009], we used 0.66, 0.60, 0.01, 0.52, and 0.202 as rates for these five events, respectively. The first three events are conceptually the same as our most probable event calculation method. The last two events are the cure/recovery or deaths for sensitive and resistant cases. These two edges go backwards. A sensitive recovery/death event indicates an isolate's movement from a sensitive status to a cured state, which we do not observe in the graph. In this case, the isolate transforms to a position with one less sensitive case than the initial count: $(i, j) \rightarrow (i - 1, j)$. The same concept applies to a resistant recovery/death event, with one less resistant case after the event: $(i, j) \rightarrow (i, j - 1)$.

We simulate an outbreak from a single sensitive case $(1, 0)$ using the five different types of events mentioned previously. Although each cluster is simulated individually, we have simulated outbreaks consisting of a set of clusters whose sizes are determined using the infinite allele model (IAM), as described in Luciani et al. [2008]. Given an outbreak size and an estimate of the IAM parameter θ (related to mutation rate and effective population size), the IAM predicts a distribution of cluster sizes. Using the estimation of θ from Luciani et al. [2008], we have used $\theta = 40$ in our calculation process to simulate an outbreak. In the simulation process, we know exactly how many cases are present in each cluster, how many clusters are in the outbreak, and how many resistance transmission and treatment failure events occurred during this process.

The outbreak sizes of the four published datasets we have used in this research range from approximately 800 to 3500. Guided by these, we have simulated different sizes of outbreaks (300–3000). However, for simplicity, only results from outbreak sizes of 300 and 1500 are shown in Figure 3.7. Once we count exactly how many events of each type occur during the simulation, the next step is taking a sample from the simulated outbreak. We use different sampling proportions, with a sampling proportion of 1 (complete sampling), 0.5, and 0.25, shown in Figure 3.7. To account for sampling, we scale up each sample using the sampling factor. Then, we can calculate events using our proposed most probable event calculation method for this scaled sample. As we don't have any genotypic information for this process, for simplicity, we assume that the source of each cluster is a single sensitive case (1, 0).

Once we have the number of each event, we can calculate the proportion of resistant events arising through transmission using both methods (simulation and proposed). Figure 3.7 shows these proportions for two different methods plotted against each other. These figures were produced for an infected outbreak size of 300 (a to c) and 1500 (d to f). We have also simulated other outbreak sizes, such as an outbreak size of 3000. The correlation between the simulated and estimated transmission proportion from an outbreak size of 3000 is very similar to the results from an outbreak size of 1500. Therefore, we have omitted the results from outbreak size 3000. These outbreaks shown in the graph include sampled and non-sampled infections. We have compared these simulated outbreaks with our estimated proportion 100 times for each outbreak size. These graphs show that when the sampling proportion is not small (approximately bigger than 0.3), the proposed method and simulation result shows a linear relationship, and they are very close to each other.

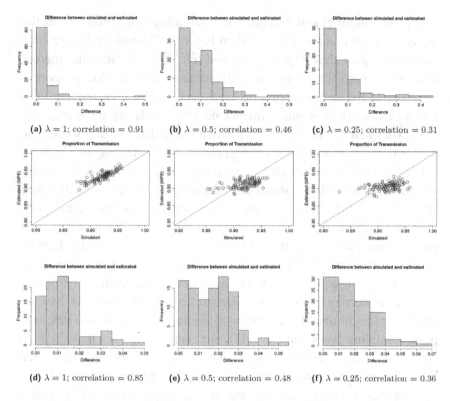

(a) $\lambda = 1$; correlation $= 0.91$ (b) $\lambda = 0.5$; correlation $= 0.46$ (c) $\lambda = 0.25$; correlation $= 0.31$

(d) $\lambda = 1$; correlation $= 0.85$ (e) $\lambda = 0.5$; correlation $= 0.48$ (f) $\lambda = 0.25$; correlation $= 0.36$

FIGURE 3.7 Comparison of the proportion of resistance due to transmission (first and third row) and the difference (second and fourth row) between simulated and estimated method is shown in the sets A to F. Three different sampling proportions ($\lambda = 1, 0.5, 0.25$) are used for each parameter (transmission proportion and difference). These graphs were produced for outbreak sizes of 300 (a to c) and 1500 (d to f—zoomed graph).

The larger outbreak size (outbreak size 1500, Figure 3.7, d to f) shows a smaller difference between simulated and estimated proportions for all different sampling proportions. However, for outbreak sizes 1500 and higher, both simulated and estimated transmission proportions usually stay between 0.8 and 1.0. Therefore, obtaining an estimated proportion within 0.05 of the simulated proportion doesn't necessarily indicate the accuracy of the method. When we look at the correlation between simulated and estimated transmission proportion in these graphs, we can see that the correlation is highest when the sampling proportion (λ) is 1 (complete sampling) and decreases with sampling proportion (correlation of Figure 3.7(a) and (d) is higher than Figure 3.7(b) and (e); Figure 3.7(b) and (e) is higher than Figure 3.7(c) and (f)). This indicates that the correlation between the simulated and estimated transmission proportion increases as the sampling proportion increases. However, the size of an outbreak doesn't have much impact on the correlation parameter. The only case when it can be an issue is when the outbreak size is small; also, the sampling proportion is small (approximately ≤ 300, Figure 3.7(c)) and is less than 0.3. The estimated transmission proportion still shows a linear relationship with the simulated proportion (correlation coefficient is approximately 0.3); however, some of the values are overestimated in the proposed MPE method. This comparison of the simulation and the proposed method shows that the MPE method is a reasonable estimate of the number of different events when the sampling proportion is not too low.

The weighting process can have an impact on estimating MPE parameters. To understand this, we will discuss an example where we have ten resistant cases in one of the clusters in the sample, and we use 10% sampling (sampling proportion $\lambda = 0.1$); our method assumes that there are 100 resistant cases in the outbreak when we account for scale-up correction. The proportion of resistance arising through transmission is 0.99 for this cluster. However, if we assume the sampling proportion is 50%, the proportion of resistance due to transmission comes down to 95%. Therefore, in the sampling process, we lose some information, and as the sampling proportion decreases, the proportion of resistance due to transmission increases. However, bigger outbreak sizes produce an exceedingly high proportion of resistance due to transmission (close to 1); scaling up does not affect these cases much.

As the outbreak sizes increase, both simulated and estimated transmission proportion increases. This is much more apparent for bigger outbreak sizes, as only a few treatment failure events (one for each cluster) are counted in the whole outbreak using the MPE method. The MPE estimate of transmission proportion $((j - 1)/j)$ clearly approaches 1 with increasing outbreak sizes. This high proportion of resistance due to transmission also reflects the simulation and real outbreaks as the parameter for transmission rate is 0.6 vs the treatment failure rate is 0.01. These parameters were estimated from real data [Tanaka et al., 2006]. As the rate of transmission is much higher than the rate of evolution (treatment failure), as the outbreak grows, the proportion will get close to 1.

Figure 3.8 shows the heat map with contour lines of the correlation and difference between the simulated and estimated transmission proportions. Here, the black contour line follows when there is an equal correlation (Figure 3.8(A)) or difference (Figure 8(B)) between the simulated and estimated transmission proportion. That is, the parameter (correlation coefficient or difference between simulated and estimated proportion) stays constant for each contour line. The contour lines from Figure 3.8(A) indicate that as the outbreak size increases, the correlation between simulated and estimated proportion due to transmission slightly decreases for sampling proportions lower than 0.6. However, there is no significant change in correlation at each level of the graph. From this graph, we can also see that the sampling proportion and the correlation coefficient (between the simulated and estimated transmission proportion) have a positive relationship. As the sampling proportion increases, the correlation between the simulated and estimated proportion (due to transmission) also increases (goes from light yellow to dark red). A high correlation coefficient indicates a good MPE transmission prediction compared to simulated outbreaks. The correlation contour plot shows that the correlation between simulated and estimated proportions is more than 0.5 if the sampling proportion is above 50%. As the colour darkens vertically, not horizontally, this indicates that the correlation coefficient is mostly dependent on the sampling proportion of the outbreak.

Figure 3.8(B) shows that the absolute difference between the simulated and estimated transmission proportion decreases as the sampling proportion increases. Here, the black contour line follows when there is an equal difference between the simulated and estimated transmission proportion. From this graph, we can see that the difference decreases as both the sampling proportion and outbreak size increase (colour lightens vertically and horizontally). Generally, the smaller the difference between the estimated and simulated transmission proportions is, the better the MPE estimate is. The absolute difference between the simulated and estimated proportion is less than 5% as long as the outbreak size is bigger than 400. Generally, it is reasonable to assume that the outbreak sizes are bigger than the size 400. This difference graph (Figure 3.8(B)) indicates that the estimated proportions get more accurate as the outbreak sizes increase and the sampling proportion increases. In summary, Figure 3.8 shows that the MPE predicts a reasonable estimate of the resistance proportion due to transmission.

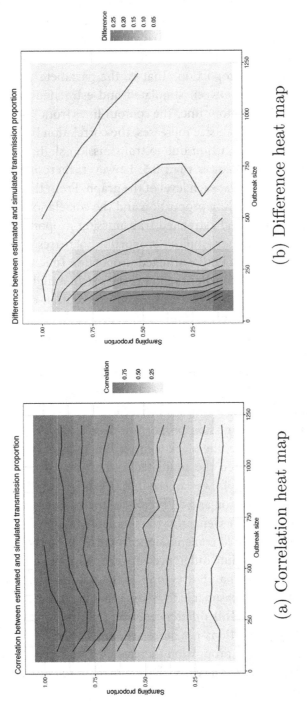

(a) Correlation heat map

(b) Difference heat map

FIGURE 3.8   Contour map comparison of the correlation (A) and difference (B) between the proportion of resistance arising through transmission using the MPE method and simulation. These graphs are produced using the average results of 3000 simulations.

3.6.2 Application to Four Datasets

We are now in a position to apply the method to published datasets to count the events in the most probable event paths leading to the observed data. These data contain resistance phenotype information for several front-line drugs, and we treat these independently so that for each drug, we classify an isolate as "sensitive" or "resistant". Therefore, these datasets contain information on drug resistance status (sensitive/resistant) for each case (people) and their genotype. Using this information, we first develop a spoligoforest. Within the spoligoforest, we assign sources for each cluster and then calculate the number of events occurring in the most probable event path of each cluster in the spoligoforest. This way, we calculate the different number of events and the proportion of resistance due to transmission/treatment failure.

We focus on the *source of resistance cases*, events T_r and A. Resistance transmission event counts for different drugs using the dataset from Monteserin et al. [2013] are shown in the second column of Table 3.2 under the assumption of complete sampling (assuming the sample represents the whole outbreak). This table shows the number of transmission events (T_r) and the proportion of resistance due to transmission (p_t). For instance, in the second column, the RIF row indicates four resistance events occur through transmission for the rifampicin drug, and the proportion of resistance due to transmission is almost 67%.

The next step is to introduce sampling proportion in this section. We calculate the proportion of resistance due to transmission (P_t) for different sampling proportions ($\lambda = 1, 0.5, 0.1, 0.01$) for all five drugs, which is shown in Table 3.2. λ is the sampling proportion, where $\lambda = 1$ indicates that the sampling proportion is 100% and we have the whole outbreak dataset sampled (complete sampling). Elaborate results of 10% sampling for each of the four different datasets are shown in Table 3.3.

Table 3.3 shows the proportion of drug resistance due to transmission (T_r) or treatment failure (A) for each drug in each dataset, assuming the sampling proportion is 10%. For instance, we can see that 93% of drug resistance to rifampicin was caused by transmission, which means 7% of resistance was caused by evolution in Diaz et al. [1998] data. The combined result shows that, on average, almost 94% of the resistance was caused by transmission (the last column in Table 3.2). Luciani et al. [2009] estimate the median of the proportion of resistance due to treatment failure to be 0.0270 [0.000, 0.238] for Cuba data and 0.019 [0.000, 0.157] for Estonia data.

TABLE 3.2 Proportion of Resistant Transmission Events Denoted by p_t for Different Sampling Proportions ($\lambda = 1, 0.5, 0.1, 0.01$). Resistant transmission events are denoted by T_r showed for five different drugs: rifampicin (RIF), isoniazid (INH), ethambutol (EMB), streptomycin (STR), and pyrazinamide (PZA). Datasets used for these calculations are collected from Monteserin et al.'s [2013] paper.

λ	1		0.5		0.1		0.01	
Drug	T_r	p_t	T_r	p_t	T_r	p_t	T_r	p_t
RIF	4	0.667	10	0.833	58	0.967	598	0.997
INH	5	0.625	13	0.813	77	0.963	797	0.996
EMB	3	0.429	10	0.714	66	0.943	696	0.994
STR	2	0.500	6	0.750	38	0.950	398	0.995
PZA	0	0	1	0.500	9	0.900	99	0.990

TABLE 3.3 Proportion of Resistant Transmission Events (P_t), Assuming That Collected Datasets Are 10% of the Whole Population. Resistant transmission events are denoted by T_r, shown for five different drugs.

	Diaz		Monteserin		Diguimbaye		Kibiki		Combined	
Drug	T_r	p_t	T_r	p_t	T_r	p_t	T_r	p_t	T_r	p_t
RIF	28	0.93	58	0.97	0	0	27	0.90	113	0.94
INH	9	0.90	77	0.96	83	0.92	101	0.92	270	0.93
EMB	0	0	66	0.94	36	0.90	27	0.90	129	0.92
STR	156	0.98	38	0.95	0	0	37	0.93	231	0.96
PZA	—	—	9	0.90	28	0.93	—	—	37	0.93

That paper estimates that > 90% of resistance cases in Estonia and Cuba are attributable to transmission, indicating that the results in Tables 3.1 and 3.2 are consistent with the findings in Luciani et al. [2009].

3.7 DISCUSSION

Our model finds the most probable events on a path and calculates different numbers of events according to the most probable event path. It shows that there is compulsorily only one evolution event in the most probable event path for each cluster, and the rest are resistant transmission events due to such a low evolution rate. We have introduced an elementary combinatorial method to estimate the proportion of drug resistance due to treatment failure. This is a significantly more efficient method than others, such as ABC [Luciani et al., 2009], and it recovers similar estimates. Compared with the simulation, the MPE estimates are very close to the actual proportions. Only smaller outbreaks with a small sampling proportion overestimate this parameter. The possible reason for overestimation is explained in section 3.6.1. However, it is reasonable to assume that the outbreak sizes are not very small when an outbreak occurs in an area.

Table 3.3 shows the result for the proportion of transmission and treatment failure events assuming a 10% sampling proportion. This table gives a clear understanding of the percentage-wise result for resistance due to transmission (p_t). Our model estimates that more than 90% of the resistance arises through transmission for all four different datasets for each drug separately, and on average, 94% of the resistance is due to transmission for all the drugs when we combine four datasets results, assuming the sampling proportion is 10%. Estimating an overall standard sampling proportion can be done by looking at estimates of overall disease load from the WHO for a region, compared to the sample sizes in the studies, as done in Tanaka et al. [2006]. However, this study is focused on estimating the relative contribution of TB transmission to the spread of resistance for different sampling proportions and does not claim that a particular sampling proportion is more common. Our result agrees with the conclusions of other studies that tuberculosis drug resistance reported in these studies arises mainly through transmission.

This chapter provides a way to estimate the proportion of drug-resistant cases that arise through transmission or treatment failure in a computationally simple way. In contrast to other methods, notably, the approximate Bayesian computation method takes days to compute. This approach does not require simulation but can be calculated from standard genotype data together with information about the resistance of individual isolates. Methods such as these should help public health bodies to make inferences about their data in a timely manner.

Increasingly, major decisions about the diagnosis and treatment of diseases are taken with the help of data-driven science. This chapter provides an efficient computational method with graph visualisation to estimate the relative contribution of transmission to the spread of TB drug resistance. This model will help understand and improve the actionable steps required to support TB disease control in real environments.

The logical next step is to examine multiple drug resistance. So far, we have looked at only single drug resistance for any isolate for simplicity. Therefore, if an isolate is resistant to any drug, we mark that isolate with a drug-resistant phenotype. However, we plan to investigate multiple drug resistance and their relationship to each other in the future. The MPE method loses some information throughout the process; however, it is a quick and practical solution. Therefore, we also plan to calculate the expected number of different events in a cluster/outbreak, considering all of the possible paths toward the final cluster. This approach will use more information about the underlying process by integrating all paths.

ACKNOWLEDGEMENTS

The authors thank Arthur Street, Natalia Vaudagnotto, Sangeeta Bhatia, and Zach Aandahl for helping develop and implement the representation of drug resistance profiles used in Figure 3.2 while their study [Aandahl et al., 2020] was in development.

REFERENCES

R Zach Aandahl, Sangeeta Bhatia, Natalia Vaudagnotto, Arthur G Street, Andrew R Francis, and Mark M Tanaka. MERCAT: Visualising molecular epidemiology data combining genetic markers and drug resistance profiles. *Infection, Genetics and Evolution*, 77:104043, 2020.

R Diaz, K Kremer, PEW De Haas, RI Gomez, A Marrero, JA Valdivia, JDA Van Embden, and D Van Soolingen. Molecular epidemiology of tuberculosis in Cuba outside of Havana, July 1994–June 1995: Utility of spoligotyping versus IS*6110* restriction fragment length polymorphism. *The International Journal of Tuberculosis and Lung Disease*, 2(9):743–750, 1998.

Colette Diguimbaye, Markus Hilty, Richard Ngandolo, Hassane H Mahamat, Gaby E Pfyffer, Franca Baggi, Marcel Tanner, Esther Schelling, and Jakob Zinsstag. Molecular characterization and drug resistance testing of *Mycobacterium tuberculosis* isolates from Chad. *Journal of Clinical Microbiology*, 44(4):1575–1577, 2006.

B Diriba, T Berkessa, G Mamo, Y Tedla, and G Ameni. Spoligotyping of multidrug resistant *Mycobacterium tuberculosis* isolates in Ethiopia. *The International Journal of Tuberculosis and Lung Disease*, 17(2):246–250, 2013.

Marcos A Espinal. The global situation of MDR-TB. *Tuberculosis*, 83(1–3):44–51, 2003.

Dorian Feldman and Martin Fox. Estimation of the parameter n in the binomial distribution. *Journal of the American Statistical Association*, 63(321):150–158, 1968.

Judith Kamerbeek, Leo Schouls, Arend Kolk, Miranda Van Agterveld, Dick Van Soolingen, Sjoukje Kuijper, Annelies Bunschoten, Henri Molhuizen, Rory Shaw, Madhu Goyal, et al. Simultaneous detection and strain differentiation of *Mycobacterium tuberculosis* for diagnosis and epidemiology. *Journal of Clinical Microbiology*, 35(4):907–914, 1997.

Gibson S Kibiki, Bert Mulder, Wil MV Dolmans, Jessica L de Beer, Martin Boeree, Noel Sam, Dick van Soolingen, Christophe Sola, and Adri GM van der Zanden. *M. tuberculosis* genotypic diversity and drug susceptibility pattern in HIV-infected and non-HIV-infected patients in northern Tanzania. *BMC Microbiology*, 1(51), 2007.

Fabio Luciani, Andrew R Francis, and Mark M Tanaka. Interpreting genotype cluster sizes of *Mycobacterium tuberculosis* isolates typed with *IS6110* and spoligotyping. *Infection, Genetics and Evolution*, 8(2):182–190, 2008.

Fabio Luciani, Scott A Sisson, Honglin Jiang, Andrew R Francis, and Mark M Tanaka. The epidemiological fitness cost of drug resistance in *Mycobacterium tuberculosis*. *Proceedings of the National Academy of Sciences*, 106(34):14711–14715, 2009.

Johana Monteserin, Mirtha Camacho, Lucía Barrera, Juan Carlos Palomino, Viviana Ritacco, and Anandi Martin. Genotypes of *Mycobacterium tuberculosis* in patients at risk of drug resistance in Bolivia. *Infection, Genetics and Evolution*, 17:195–201, 2013.

Cagri Ozcaglar, Amina Shabbeer, Scott L Vandenberg, Bülent Yener, and Kristin P Bennett. Epidemiological models of *Mycobacterium tuberculosis* complex infections. *Mathematical Biosciences*, 236(2):77–96, 2012.

Josephine F Reyes, Andrew R Francis, and Mark M Tanaka. Models of deletion for visualizing bacterial variation: An application to tuberculosis spoligotypes. *BMC Bioinformatics*, 9(1):496, 2008.

Josephine F Reyes, Carmen HS Chan, and Mark M Tanaka. Impact of homoplasy on variable numbers of tandem repeats and spoligotypes in *Mycobacterium tuberculosis*. *Infection, Genetics and Evolution*, 12(4):811–818, 2012.

Guilherme S Rodrigues, Andrew R Francis, Scott A Sisson, and Mark M Tanaka. Inferences on the acquisition of multi-drug resistance in mycobacterium tuberculosis using molecular epidemiological data. In *Handbook of Approximate Bayesian Computation*, pp. 481–511. Chapman and Hall/CRC, 2018.

EM Streicher, TC Victor, G Van Der Spuy, C Sola, N Rastogi, PD Van Helden, and RM Warren. Spoligotype signatures in the *Mycobacterium tuberculosis* complex. *Journal of Clinical Microbiology*, 45(1):237–240, 2007.

Mark M Tanaka, Andrew R Francis, Fabio Luciani, and SA Sisson. Using approximate Bayesian computation to estimate tuberculosis transmission parameters from genotype data. *Genetics*, 173(3):1511–1520, 2006.

WHO. Who 2020. www.who.int/news-room/fact-sheets/detail/tuberculosis, 2020.

A Wright, G Bai, L Barrera, F Boulahbal, N Martin-Casabona, C Gilpin, F Drobniewski, M Havelkov´a, R Lepe, R Lumb, et al. Emergence of mycobacterium tuberculosis with extensive resistance to second-line drugs—Worldwide, 2000–2004. *Morbidity and Mortality Weekly Report*, 55(11):301–306, 2006.

A Novel Diagnosis System for Parkinson's Disease Based on Ensemble Random Forest

Arkadip Ray and Avijit Kumar Chaudhuri

4.1 INTRODUCTION

Parkinson's disease (PD) is a serious health problem that affects millions of individuals worldwide. This is a prototypical adult-onset neurodegenerative disorder originally described by Doctor James Parkinson as shaking palsy [1]. The patient's health deteriorates over time as a result of this chronic illness. Many motor and non-motor processes in the human body are regulated by dopamine, a neurotransmitter produced by neurons in the biological neural network. Certain cell body clusters in PD neurons are unable to generate dopamine. The amount of dopamine produced in the neurological system decreases as PD progresses, causing a person to become incapable of moving appropriately [2, 3]. In the early stages of Parkinson's disease, tremors in one hand, foot, or leg are often the first signs and symptoms. Slow movement, stiffness, decreased body balance, difficulty in standing, decreased facial expressions, coordination issues, difficulty in thinking, difficulty in understanding, difficulty in writing, distorted sense of smell, dribbling urine, impaired voice, soft speech, and voice box spasms are some of the other symptoms [2–5]. In 90% of these

DOI: 10.1201/9781003292357-4

cases, the individual has vocal dysfunction, making it difficult to speak or communicate [6]. Using modern signal processing algorithms, doctors can diagnose and track the progress of the disease by carefully examining the sound and voice of PD patients.

The absence of any known risk factors makes diagnosis especially difficult, and consistency of results between doctors is difficult. Based on risk factors, it is difficult to determine the risk of PD or make a diagnosis [7]. The machine learning approach is beneficial in this scenario because it provides insights and reveals patterns based on improved data collection, storage, and processing capabilities. By using machine learning techniques, PD risk can be predicted early on. Any error in disease prediction, especially Type II errors, has the potential to be fatal. In addition to accuracy, other performance measures such as consistency, sensitivity, and specificity are relevant in such studies. Several machine learning techniques for disease prediction in general, and PD in particular, fail to meet these additional performance criteria.

We introduce a novel ensemble random forest (ERF) classifier in this paper. It is compared against many cutting-edge machine learning classifiers like logistic regression (LR), naïve Bayes (NB), decision tree (DT), support vector machine (SVM), and random forest (RF), as well as earlier research on the same dataset. Several performance measures (accuracy, sensitivity, specificity, receiver operating characteristic (ROC), area under the curve (AUC), kappa statistic) are compared on 50–50%, 66–34%, and 80–20% splits of training and testing data and a 20-fold cross-validation.

In this study, we aim to answer the following research questions:

- Research Question 1: Is the suggested ERF classifier suitable for PD prediction?

- Research Question 2: Does the suggested ERF classifier fulfill the added sensitivity and specificity criteria?

- Research Question 3: Is the suggested ERF classifier consistent and statistically significant throughout the dataset's various levels of training and testing samples?

A flowchart of experimental design and model construction is shown in Figure 4.1.

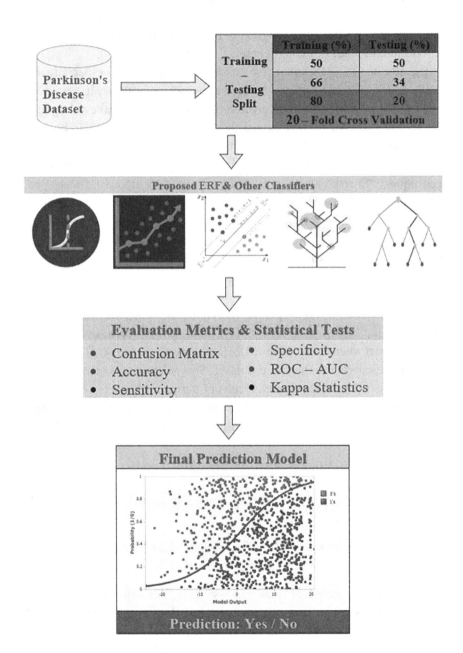

FIGURE 4.1 PD prediction model.

4.2 RELATED WORK

The development of advanced diagnostic and detection technologies for disease is becoming possible with technological advancements [8]. In practically every area of medicine, researchers have used machine learning, expert systems, and soft computing approaches [9, 10]. Various ways of diagnosing PD are available in the literature through adequate modeling of voice and speech datasets. Preprocessing, feature extraction, and classification are critical phases of these computerized classification systems. Using a kernel support vector machine with a feature selection approach, Little et al. [11] accurately diagnosed PD with 91.4% accuracy. Nonlinear models using Dirichlet process mixtures for PD diagnosis have been proposed by Little et al. [11], Shahbaba and Neal [12], and Psorakis et al. [13]. The authors [12] employed improved multi-class multi-kernel relevance vector machines (mRVMs) and attained 89.47% with the ten-fold cross-validation approach. Psorakis et al. [13] suggested a model based on genetic programming and the expectation-maximization technique. Guo et al. [14], Psorakis et al. [13], and Sakar and Kursun [15] built an appropriate model based on the mutual information measure and support vector machines. Sakar and Kursun [15] and Das [16] conducted a comparative analysis of four separate classification models and found that the artificial neural network–based model had the highest accuracy (92.9%). Das [16] and Luukka [17] used fuzzy entropy metrics and a similarity classifier. This study produced an average actual accuracy of 85.03% using a 50/50 training and testing set. For the diagnosis of PD, Luukka [17] and Ozcift and Gulten [18] suggested a correlation-based feature selection (CFS) technique with rotating forest ensemble classifiers. To improve classification performance on relatively small datasets, Ozcift and Gulten [18] and Li et al. [19] presented fuzzy-based nonlinear transformation approaches using principal component analysis (PCA) and SVM. To demonstrate the performance of their technique, they applied it to six medical datasets, including a PD dataset.

Using parallel artificial neural network architecture, Astrom and Koker [20] achieved 91.20% classification accuracy. Spadoto et al. [21] used evolutionary-based feature selection strategies to increase the accuracy of an optimum path forest classifier for PD diagnosis. Polat [22] applied a fuzzy c-means (FCM) clustering-based feature weighting approach and a K-nearest neighbor (KNN) classifier to yield a 97.93%

accuracy rate. An accuracy of 91.20% was achieved with a chi-square kernel SVM developed by Daliri [23]. Based on PCA and fuzzy KNN, Chen et al. [24] achieved 96.07% accuracy with ten-fold cross-validation. Zuo et al. [25] used an evolutionary approach (particle swarm optimization) to improve the performance of a fuzzy k-nearest neighbor classifier, resulting in an accuracy of 97.47%. Zhang [26] presented PD diagnosis utilizing time-frequency characteristics, stacked autoencoders (SAEs), and KNN classifiers.

4.3 METHODOLOGY

4.3.1 Dataset

As part of a collaboration between the National Centre for Voice and Speech in Denver, Colorado, and Max Little of the University of Oxford, speech signals were collected in the dataset. The feature extraction approaches for general voice problems were reported in the original paper. The PD study dataset contains biomedical voice measurements from 31 patients, 23 of whom have Parkinson's disease. In the table, each column represents a distinct voice measure, and each row represents one of the 195 recordings ("name" column) of each person, as depicted in Table 4.1. Using the "status" column, which is set to 0 for healthy people and 1 for those with PD, the data are primarily designed to distinguish between the two groups [27]. Data are stored in ASCII comma-separated values (CSV) format, with each row representing a single voice recording instance. For each patient, there are approximately six recordings, with the patient's name in the first column.

4.3.2 Algorithm for the ERF and Stacking

Suppose we are considering a set of training data $\left\{\left(x_j, y_j\right)\right\}_{j=1}^{K}$, where $x_j \in R^Q$ and $y_j \in \{-1,1\}$, and suppose we are given a potentially large number of logistic regression classifiers as weak classifiers, denoted $f_p(x) \in \{-1,1\}$, and a 0–1 loss function I, defined as

$$I\left(f_m(a), b\right) = \begin{cases} 0 \text{ if }_m\left(a_i\right) = b_i \\ 0 \text{ if }_m\left(a_i\right) \neq b_i \end{cases}$$

Then the algorithm of the AdaBoost can be illustrated as follows.

TABLE 4.1   Description of PD Study Dataset

Order No	Attributes	Description	Range of Values	Mean	Standard Deviation
1	name	Patient name in ASCII and recording number	—	—	—
2	MDVP: Fo (Hz)	Vocal fundamental frequency on average	88.333–260.105	154.228641	41.39006475
3	MDVP: Fhi (Hz)	Maximum fundamental frequency of the voice	102.145–592.03	197.1049179	91.49154764
4	MDVP: Flo (Hz)	Minimum fundamental frequency of the voice	65.476–239.17	116.3246308	43.52141318
5	MDVP: Jitter (%)	Several measures of fundamental frequency variation	0.00168–0.03316	0.00622	0.004848
6	MDVP: Jitter (Abs)		0.000007–0.00026	4.40E-05	3.48E-05
7	MDVP: RAP		0.00068–0.02144	0.00330641	0.002967774
8	MDVP: PPQ		0.00092–0.01958	0.003446359	0.002758977
9	Jitter: DDP		0.00204–0.06433	0.009919949	0.008903344
10	MDVP: Shimmer	Several amplitude variations	0.00954–0.11908	0.029709128	0.018856932
11	MDVP: Shimmer (dB)		0.085–1.302	0.282251282	0.19487729
12	Shimmer: APQ3		0.00455–0.05647	0.015664154	0.010153162
13	Shimmer: APQ5		0.0057–0.0794	0.017878256	0.012023706
14	MDVP: APQ		0.00719–0.13778	0.024081487	0.016946736
15	Shimmer: DDA		0.01364–0.16942	0.046992615	0.030459119

(Continued)

TABLE 4.1   (Continued)

Order No	Attributes	Description	Range of Values	Mean	Standard Deviation
16	NHR	Two measurements of the	0.00065–0.31482	0.024847077	0.040418449
17	HNR	noise-to-tonal component ratio in the voice	8.441–33.047	21.88597436	4.425764269
18	RPDE	There are two measurements	0.25657–0.685151	0.498535538	0.103941714
19	D2	of nonlinear dynamical complexity	1.423287–3.671155	2.381826087	0.382799047
20	DFA	Exponent of signal fractal scaling	0.574282 —0.825288	0.718099046	0.05533583
21	spread1	Three nonlinear measurements	(−7.964984)–(−2.434031)	−5.684396744	1.090207764
22	spread2	of fundamental frequency	0.006274–0.450493	0.226510349	0.083405763
23	PPE	fluctuation	0.044539–0.527367	0.206551641	0.090119322
24	status	Patients' health conditions 1: PD 0: healthy			

$$\text{for } j \text{ from 1 to } N, w_j^{(J)} = 1$$

$$\text{for } m = 1 \text{ to } M \text{ do}$$

Fit weak classifier m (random forest) to minimize the objective function:

$$\epsilon_m = \frac{\sum_{j=1}^{N} w_j^{(m)} I\left(f_x\left(a_j\right) \neq b_j\right)}{\sum_j w_j^{(m)}}$$

where $I\left(f_p\left(a_j\right) \neq b_j\right) = 1$ if $f_p\left(a_j\right) \neq b_j$ and 0 otherwise

$$\alpha_m = \ln \frac{1 - \epsilon_m}{\epsilon_m}$$

for all j do

$$w_j^{(m+1)} = w_j^{(m)} e^{\alpha_m I\left(f_p\left(x_j\right) \neq y_j\right)}$$

end for

end for

After learning, the final classifier is based on a linear combination of the logistic regressions: $g(x) = \text{sign}\left(\sum_{m=1}^{M} \alpha_m f_m(x)\right)$

4.4 RESULTS AND DISCUSSION

Using the Python programming language, the authors developed and simulated a model. A comparative study was conducted with the proposed model and five state-of-the-art machine learning algorithms, LR, RF, NB, SVM, and DT. These five popular machine learning techniques display varying levels of accuracy, with some more accurate than others. Using advanced ensemble machine learning techniques, the authors devised an ensemble meta-algorithm technique to improve the weak classifier's accuracy and performance (Figure 4.2).

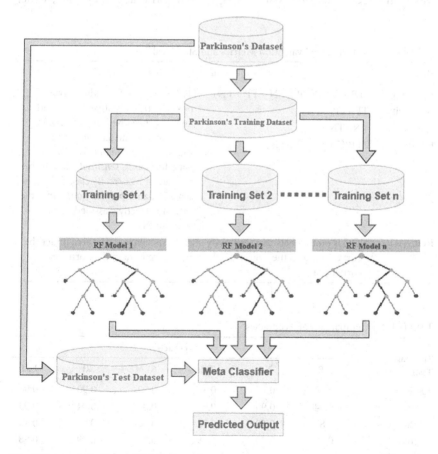

FIGURE 4.2   Working of ERF classifier.

This experiment is designed to classify healthy people and people with Parkinson's disease. This purpose was achieved by applying machine learning techniques to the UCI dataset of biomedical voice measurements called Oxford Parkinson's Disease Detection (OPD). Table 4.2 presents the performance evaluation matrices used in this study. A review of Table 4.3 shows that different approaches yield different accuracy levels, with NB recording an accuracy rate of 70%, while the proposed ERF measured 96%.

A confusion matrix presents the statistics of real and projected classifications achieved from the analysis of different classification systems. The performance of all such systems is generally assessed using the data generated in this matrix. Table 4.4 shows the results generated from confusion matrices using different machine learning algorithms. The performance of the proposed model, along with the performances of other methods, was evaluated based on sensitivity, specificity, and accuracy tests, which

TABLE 4.2   Performance Evaluation Metrics and Statistical Tests

Metrics	Formula/Description	
Accuracy	$(TP + TN)/(TP + TN + FP + FN)$	TP, TN, FP, and FN indicate true
Sensitivity	$TP/(TP + FN)$	positive, true negative, false positive,
Specificity	$TN/(TN + FP)$	and false negative, respectively. In
F-Score	$2TP/(2TP + FP + FN)$	other words, the term *accuracy* measures the rate of correctly classified cases, *sensitivity* determines the rate of incorrectly classified cases with PD, and *specificity* quantifies the rate of correctly classified cases without PD.
ROC-AUC	ROC is plotted between sensitivity and (1- specificity). The area under the curve measures the degree to which the curve is up in the northwest corner [28].	

TABLE 4.3   Comparison of Accuracies

Training–Testing Split	Accuracies					
	LR	NB	DT	SVM	RF	ERF
50–50	0.90	0.75	0.86	0.92	0.90	0.96
66–34	0.84	0.90	0.85	0.85	0.94	0.93
80–20	0.87	0.69	0.92	0.87	0.92	0.95
20-fold cross validation	0.82	0.70	0.79	0.84	0.79	0.88

TABLE 4.4   Comparison of Sensitivity and Specificity

		Training–Testing Split			20-fold cross validation
		50–50	66–34	80–20	
LR	*Sensitivity*	0.89	0.86	0.89	0.82
	Specificity	0.93	0.75	0.75	0.85
NB	*Sensitivity*	0.96	0.92	0.92	0.70
	Specificity	0.48	0.47	0.33	0.97
DT	*Sensitivity*	0.91	0.90	0.94	0.79
	Specificity	0.70	0.71	0.83	0.87
SVM	*Sensitivity*	0.90	0.87	0.89	0.84
	Specificity	1	0.77	0.75	0.86
RF	*Sensitivity*	0.93	0.94	0.94	0.89
	Specificity	0.78	0.93	0.83	0.94
ERF	*Sensitivity*	0.96	0.94	0.94	0.88
	Specificity	0.95	0.88	1	0.87

consider the true positive (TP), true negative (TN), false negative (FN), and false positive (FP) terms.

The results of sensitivity and specificity in Table 4.4 demonstrate the potential of the conceptual model in the classification of two classes. The comparison of the proposed model with other widely used independent classification techniques is shown in Table 4.6. As can be seen from the comparative results, the proposed classification technique has the highest accuracy, sensitivity, and specificity values (accuracy = 96%, sensitivity = 0.96, specificity = 1).

A 90% classification accuracy was achieved by LR, with a sensitivity of 89% and specificity of 93%. Classification accuracy for RF was 94%, while sensitivity and specificity were both 94%. Classification accuracy by SVM was 92%, with 90% sensitivity and 100% specificity. The proposed classifier performed most effectively of the six classifiers evaluated, achieving 96% accuracy in classification, 96% sensitivity, and 100% specificity. A complete list of results can be seen in Tables 4.3 and 4.4.

Analytical results of the proposed classifier are equally acceptable. A significant outcome of the developed classifier is its enhanced specificity and sensitivity to predict PD. While NB produced 96% sensitivity and 97% specificity, the other classifiers produced lower sensitivity and specificity. Using the proposed classifier, those disadvantages were eliminated, yielding sensitivity and specificity of 96% and 100%, respectively, which indicates that fewer patients would need to be tested for PD due to improved specificity. Moreover, a higher sensitivity value would save money and minimize the waiting time for really ill patients, both of which would be crucial to lifesaving.

Researchers have studied the F-measure extensively in the context of information retrieval and class imbalance issues. The fundamental advantage of the F-measure is that it compares classifier performance in terms of recall (or true positive rate) to accuracy using a factor that adjusts their relative relevance [29]. F-measure results in Table 4.5 demonstrate the potential of the suggested model for classifying two classes. This table compares the proposed model to several commonly applied independent classification algorithms. For the PD dataset, the suggested classification algorithm produced the highest F-measure values (97%).

The AUC values derived from ROC charts for these experiments with individual machine learning techniques are depicted in Table 4.6. According to experimental results, the proposed classifier outperformed most of the previously used methods discussed in the literature review in terms of cross-validation accuracy. With the proposed model, the generated AUC value reached 0.95.

Comparisons based only on accuracy might yield ambiguous results when comparing the performances of different machine learning classifiers. The Cohen's kappa statistic (CKS) value is used to help produce error-free comparative efficiency of different classifiers [30]. In these evaluations, the cost of errors must be taken into account. In this respect, CKS is an excellent measure for inspecting classifications that may be due to chance. Usually CKS ranges between –1 and +1. As the classifier's calculated kappa value approaches 1, its performance is assumed to be more realistic than "by chance". Therefore, the CKS value is a suggested metric

TABLE 4.5   Comparison of F-Score

Training–Testing Split	F-Score					
	LR	NB	DT	SVM	RF	ERF
50–50	0.94	0.81	0.91	0.95	0.93	0.97
66–34	0.90	0.78	0.90	0.90	0.96	0.95
80–20	0.93	0.79	0.95	0.93	0.95	0.97
20-fold cross validation	0.80	0.78	0.80	0.82	0.90	0.90

TABLE 4.6　Comparison of AUC

Training–Testing Split	AUC					
	LR	NB	DT	SVM	RF	ERF
20-fold cross validation	0.84	0.82	0.73	0.80	0.93	0.95

TABLE 4.7　Kappa Statistic for Each Model

Training–Testing Split	Kappa Statistic					
	LR	NB	DT	SVM	RF	ERF
50–50	0.68	0.46	0.60	0.74	0.72	0.88
66–34	0.52	0.40	0.61	0.57	0.84	0.80
80–20	0.48	0.28	0.72	0.48	0.72	0.80
20-fold cross validation	0.40	0.48	0.43	0.45	0.70	0.66

for measurement purposes in the performance analysis of classifiers [31]. The kappa value is calculated using Equation 1.

$$CKS = \frac{PR_a - PR_{ac}}{(1 - PR_{ac})} \qquad (1)$$

where PR_a represents total agreement probability and PR_{ac} represents probability "by chance".

The results of the CKS analysis of the five popular machine learning techniques and the proposed model are shown in Table 4.7. These results demonstrate that the proposed model performed much better than other classifiers (value = 0.88).

4.5 CONCLUSION

Worldwide, PD is among the leading causes of mortality, particularly in low- and middle-income countries. A series of medical tests and their interpretation by experts are required to diagnose PD. It may be difficult to diagnose a patient when the results of medical tests differ, and it may impair the consistency of doctors' diagnoses. In this situation, machine learning techniques can identify patterns and provide insights.

TABLE 4.8   PD Dataset Performance Comparison

Literature Reference	Method	Accuracy (%)	Sensitivity/ Specificity	F-Measure	Kappa	ROC/AUC
[32]	ANFC-LH	94.72	0.88/1	×	×	×
	MLPNN	89.69	0.88/0.96	×	×	×
	RBFNN	87.63	0.88/0.96	×	×	×
[33]	PNN	81.28	×	×	×	×
[34]	GA-WK-ELM	96.81	0.95/0.98	×	×	×
[35]	CBFO-FKNN	96.97	0.97/0.99	×	×	0.98
[18]	CFS-RF	87.10	×	×	×	0.86
[36]	SVM-BFO	97.42	0.99/0.92	×	×	×
[24]	PCA-FKNN	96.07	0.96/0.96	×	×	0.96
[37]	FESA-DNN	92.19	0.97/0.90	×	×	×
This study	**ERF**	**96**	**0.96/1**	**0.97**	**0.88**	**0.95**

The suggested ensemble random forest classifier, like the stacking-ensemble approach, combines the random forest classifier predictions utilizing RF (also) as the meta-classifier. The classes in the dataset are distributed unequally. Unbalanced datasets increase the risk of misdiagnosing a sick patient as healthy (which is very severe) and decrease the likelihood of misdiagnosing a healthy patient. The proposed classifier is compared with two parametric (LR and NB) and three non-parametric classifiers (SVM with a radial basis kernel, DT, and RF). This comparison is based on accuracy, sensitivity, specificity, F-measure, ROC, AUC, and kappa statistics. The authors use 50–50%, 66–34%, and 80–20% train–test splits, as well as 20-fold cross-validation. There are no identical records of PD patients in the training and testing datasets. In general, non-parametric classifiers perform better than parametric classifiers (whose learning is limited by their assumptions), and the random forest classifier outperforms them all. With 96% accuracy and a lower false positive/negative rate, the proposed classifier outperforms random forest.

REFERENCES

1. Parkinson, J. (2002). An essay on the shaking palsy. The Journal of Neuropsychiatry and Clinical Neurosciences, 14(2), 223–236.
2. Langston, J. W. (2002). Parkinson's disease: Current and future challenges. Neurotoxicology, 23(4–5), 443–450.
3. Meissner, W. G., Frasier, M., Gasser, T., Goetz, C. G., Lozano, A., Piccini, P., . . . & Bezard, E. (2011). Priorities in Parkinson's disease research. Nature Reviews Drug Discovery, 10(5), 377–393.

4. Gallagher, D. A., Lees, A. J., & Schrag, A. (2010). What are the most important nonmotor symptoms in patients with Parkinson's disease and are we missing them? Movement Disorders, 25(15), 2493–2500.
5. Mittel, C. S. (2002). Parkinson's disease: Overview and current abstracts. 1st edition, Nova Science Pub Inc., Hauppauge, NY.
6. Schley, W. S., Fenton, E., & Niimi, S. (1982). Vocal symptoms in Parkinson disease treated with levodopa: A case report. Annals of Otology, Rhinology & Laryngology, 91(1), 119–121.
7. Akyol, K. (2017). A study on the diagnosis of Parkinson's disease using digitized Wacom graphics tablet dataset. International Journal of Computer Science and Information Technology, 9, 45–51.
8. Ray, A., & Chaudhuri, A. K. (2021). Smart healthcare disease diagnosis and patient management: Innovation, improvement and skill development. Machine Learning with Applications, 3, 100011.
9. Chaudhuri, A. K., Sinha, D., Banerjee, D. K., & Das, A. (2021a). A novel enhanced decision tree model for detecting chronic kidney disease. Network Modeling Analysis in Health Informatics and Bioinformatics, 10(1), 1–22.
10. Chaudhuri, A. K., Ray, A., Banerjee, D. K., & Das, A. (2021b). A multi-stage approach combining feature selection with machine learning techniques for higher prediction reliability and accuracy in cervical cancer diagnosis. International Journal of Intelligent Systems and Applications, 13, 46–63.
11. Little, M., McSharry, P., Hunter, E., Spielman, J., & Ramig, L. (2008). Suitability of dysphonia measurements for telemonitoring of Parkinson's disease. Nature Proceedings, 1–1.
12. Shahbaba, B., & Neal, R. (2009). Nonlinear models using Dirichlet process mixtures. Journal of Machine Learning Research, 10(8).
13. Psorakis, I., Damoulas, T., & Girolami, M. A. (2010). Multiclass relevance vector machines: Sparsity and accuracy. IEEE Transactions on Neural Networks, 21(10), 1588–1598.
14. Guo, P. F., Bhattacharya, P., & Kharma, N. (2010, June). Advances in detecting Parkinson's disease. In International Conference on Medical Biometrics (pp. 306–314). Springer, Berlin and Heidelberg.
15. Sakar, C. O., & Kursun, O. (2010). Telediagnosis of Parkinson's disease using measurements of dysphonia. Journal of Medical Systems, 34(4), 591–599.
16. Das, R. (2010). A comparison of multiple classification methods for diagnosis of Parkinson disease. Expert Systems with Applications, 37(2), 1568–1572.
17. Luukka, P. (2011). Feature selection using fuzzy entropy measures with similarity classifier. Expert Systems with Applications, 38(4), 4600–4607.
18. Ozcift, A., & Gulten, A. (2011). Classifier ensemble construction with rotation forest to improve medical diagnosis performance of machine learning algorithms. Computer Methods and Programs in Biomedicine, 104(3), 443–451.
19. Li, D. C., Liu, C. W., & Hu, S. C. (2011). A fuzzy-based data transformation for feature extraction to increase classification performance with small medical datasets. Artificial Intelligence in Medicine, 52(1), 45–52.

20. Åström, F., & Koker, R. (2011). A parallel neural network approach to prediction of Parkinson's Disease. Expert Systems with Applications, 38(10), 12470–12474.

21. Spadoto, A. A., Guido, R. C., Carnevali, F. L., Pagnin, A. F., Falcão, A. X., & Papa, J. P. (2011, August). Improving Parkinson's disease identification through evolutionary-based feature selection. In 2011 Annual International Conference of the IEEE Engineering in Medicine and Biology Society (pp. 7857–7860). IEEE, New York.

22. Polat, K. (2012). Classification of Parkinson's disease using feature weighting method on the basis of fuzzy C-means clustering. International Journal of Systems Science, 43(4), 597–609.

23. Daliri, M. R. (2013). Chi-square distance kernel of the gaits for the diagnosis of Parkinson's disease. Biomedical Signal Processing and Control, 8(1), 66–70.

24. Chen, H. L., Huang, C. C., Yu, X. G., Xu, X., Sun, X., Wang, G., & Wang, S. J. (2013). An efficient diagnosis system for detection of Parkinson's disease using fuzzy k-nearest neighbor approach. Expert Systems with Applications, 40(1), 263–271.

25. Zuo, W. L., Wang, Z. Y., Liu, T., & Chen, H. L. (2013). Effective detection of Parkinson's disease using an adaptive fuzzy k-nearest neighbor approach. Biomedical Signal Processing and Control, 8(4), 364–373.

26. Zhang, Y. N. (2017). Can a smartphone diagnose Parkinson disease? A deep neural network method and telediagnosis system implementation. Parkinson's Disease, 2017, 6209703.

27. Little, M., Mcsharry, P., Roberts, S., Costello, D., & Moroz, I. (2007). Exploiting nonlinear recurrence and fractal scaling properties for voice disorder detection. Nature Proceedings, 1–1.

28. Vandewiele, G., Dehaene, I., Kovács, G., Sterckx, L., Janssens, O., Ongenae, F., . . . & Demeester, T. (2021). Overly optimistic prediction results on imbalanced data: A case study of flaws and benefits when applying over-sampling. Artificial Intelligence in Medicine, 111, 101987.

29. Soleymani, R., Granger, E., & Fumera, G. (2020). F-measure curves: A tool to visualize classifier performance under imbalance. Pattern Recognition, 100, 107146.

30. Chaudhuri, A. K., Banerjee, D. K., & Das, A. (2021). A dataset centric feature selection and stacked model to detect breast cancer. International Journal of Intelligent Systems and Applications (IJISA), 13(4), 24–37.

31. Ben-David, A. (2008). Comparison of classification accuracy using Cohen's weighted kappa. Expert Systems with Applications, 34(2), 825–832.

32. Çağlar, M. F., Çetişli, B., & Toprak, I. B. (2010). Automatic recognition of Parkinson's disease from sustained phonation tests using ANN and adaptive neuro-fuzzy classifier. Mühendislik Bilimleri ve Tasarım Dergisi, 1(2), 59–64.

33. Ene, M. (2008). Neural network-based approach to discriminate healthy people from those with Parkinson's disease. Annals of the University of Craiova-Mathematics and Computer Science Series, 35, 112–116.

34. Avci, D., & Dogantekin, A. (2016). An expert diagnosis system for Parkinson disease based on genetic algorithm-wavelet kernel-extreme learning machine. Parkinson's Disease, 2016.
35. Cai, Z., Gu, J., Wen, C., Zhao, D., Huang, C., Huang, H., . . . & Chen, H. (2018). An intelligent Parkinson's disease diagnostic system based on a chaotic bacterial foraging optimization enhanced fuzzy KNN approach. Computational and Mathematical Methods in Medicine, 2018.
36. Cai, Z., Gu, J., & Chen, H. L. (2017). A new hybrid intelligent framework for predicting Parkinson's disease. IEEE Access, 5, 17188–17200.
37. Kadam, V. J., & Jadhav, S. M. (2019). Feature ensemble learning based on sparse autoencoders for diagnosis of Parkinson's disease. In Computing, Communication and Signal Processing (pp. 567–581). Springer.

CHAPTER 5

Harmonization of Brain Data across Sites and Scanners

Ilias Aitterrami, Edouard Duchesnay,
and Carol Anne Hargreaves

5.1 INTRODUCTION

5.1.1 Background

Medical studies, especially those focusing on images, are based on small dataset sizes, because they usually require follow-up on patients for many months or years, which is very demanding. Multi-site studies provide the opportunity to have access to more data and allow more follow-up of patients; hence, more information about disease behavior and treatment efficiency is captured.

The main issue observed with multi-site studies, particularly with magnetic resonance imaging (MRI) studies, is the non-biological variability existing in the measures, which is mainly due to the use of different scanners or parameter configurations. The use of different scanners can also be a consequence of social inequalities for different hospital regions or other local parameters. Also, since we do not have any information about patient income, for example, or any other social indicators in the datasets, we have focused on general inter-site variability without differentiating what might be due to scanners and what might be due to other aspects. We define the term harmonization process as the explicit removal of site-related effects in multi-site data. The research conducted in this work is mainly a benchmark of existing harmonization methods and a discussion of the existing methods.

DOI: 10.1201/9781003292357-5

We briefly provide the benefit of using machine learning and deep learning in MRI to better understand why it is critical to have reliable datasets. The use of machine learning and deep learning is commonly called artificial intelligence (AI). AI has led to unprecedented advances in the medical field, with applications in risk assessment, diagnosis, prediction of treatment effectiveness, and brain imaging in the understanding of strokes, psychopathic or degenerative disorders, diseases such as epilepsy whose origin and evolution are still difficult to understand, and many others. MRI brain data are difficult to obtain and interpret. We demonstrate through a few examples the use of MRI brain data and interpret the results. Being able to conduct multi-site brain image studies is a major issue due to the scarcity of the images and the shortage of AI talent to interpret the brain image patterns. Hence, this study is valuable and contributes greatly to the brain MRI image research area.

5.1.2 Research Objective

The objective of this study is to find a robust harmonization method that removes inter-site variability while preserving the biological variability of brain MRI image data. We aim to:

- Build a fixed effects model to identify an additive site effect using a linear regression model,

- Build an adjusted linear regression model, where we include age and sex biological features in the model,

- Build a random effects model, that is, a ComBat model, using an additive and multiplicative site effect, and

- Discuss how these three traditional harmonization methods are evaluated in previous work and propose a slightly different way of evaluating the models that reduces the impact of a potential bias in the results presented.

This chapter is organized into five sections. Section 5.2 is a literature review mainly introducing the three harmonization methods we will focus on. Section 5.3 is a description of the proposed methodology. Section 5.4 presents the results and discussion, and the conclusion is covered in Section 5.5.

5.2 LITERATURE REVIEW

Artificial intelligence is a research tool that opens the door to enormous progress in a multitude of fields, provided that the data used or collected to conduct the studies are exploitable. The field of AI applications is very varied; the medical field in particular interests us here, but there are also AI applications in marketing, education, law, and business. Many academicians consider artificial intelligence the future of society [1]. There is a growing need for reliable data, especially in areas such as medicine, where people's lives are at stake. The harmonization of multi-site data is therefore a major challenge to take advantage of the new methods offered by artificial intelligence.

We will refer to the process of removing site effects as harmonization of the data and will refer to the data after harmonization as residualized or harmonized data. The type of data handled in this work will vary, giving different information each time about the patient's brain. For this part, let's consider that we manipulate average volumes of grey matter of regions of interest of the brain (a region of interest, or ROI, will be defined later). We first go through the fixed effect model, where we identify an additive site effect through a rather basic linear regression model. We next look at a random effect model (ComBat), complexifying a bit of the previous models with an additive and a multiplicative site effect and presenting, according to the literature, several advantages. The first residualization or harmonization method is a very simple linear regression model. The idea is to model the site effect within a predictor in the regression and then subtract it from the initial data [2]. For now, we do not consider any other covariates in the regression model. One-hot encoding was used to convert the categorical variables, in our case the site information, in a $n \times p$ matrix with an intercept and $p \times 1$ columns, where p is the number of sites. Thanks to one-hot encoding, categorical variables can be taken into consideration in regression models, where each site is represented by a zero and one column, except for one that is represented by the intercept and all other columns.

The linear regression model is as follows:

$$X_i = \alpha_i + Z_{site}\beta_i + \epsilon_i \tag{1}$$

where $\mathbf{X_i}$ is a $n \times 1$ vector whose coefficients correspond to the average volume of grey matter of the ROI, i for each subject, α_i is the average volume of the ROI, i for the reference site, written as a constant $n \times 1$–column vector, Z_{site} is the design matrix of the regression model, which is for this first model the one-hot encoding of the site information, β_i and is the $p \times 1$ parameter vector of the regression model for the ROI$_i$, which is estimated using the ordinary least squares (OLS) method, and ϵ_i is the $n \times 1$ residual term with an expected value of zero. Note that we used an unusual X notation for the output because we are presenting the harmonization methods of the features of interest, which were used after harmonization to conduct the studies. We prefer to keep the X notation from the beginning to avoid any misunderstanding.

To be closer to the literature, we can also write the non-vectorized version of the regression model as follows:

$$X_{ijk} = \alpha_i + \gamma_{ik} + \epsilon_{ikj} \tag{2}$$

where X_{ikj} is the average volume of grey matter of the ROI i for subject j coming from site k; α_i is the average volume of the ROI i (just a scalar this time); γ_{ik} is the coefficient of $Z_{site}\beta_i$ corresponding to site k; and ϵ_{ikj} is the residual term (for ROI i, site k, and subject j) with an expected value of zero [6].

Once the additive site effect is estimated, the volumes are residualized as follows:

$$X_i^{\sim res} = X_i - Z_{site}\hat{\beta}_i \tag{3}$$

where $\hat{\beta}^i$ is the OLS estimator of β_i. Or as follows:

$$X_{ikj}^{\sim res} = X_{ikj} + \hat{y}_{ik} \tag{4}$$

where $\hat{y}_{ik}$ is the OLS estimator of γ_{ik}.

By subtracting the site coefficient of the linear regression model, the fixed additive site effect on the volumes is removed.

The term "non-adjusted" in the previous model refers to the fact that the harmonization is not adjusted on covariables of interest such as age or sex of the subject, and this is problematic because important information can be lost through the harmonization, while we only want to remove the site variability. In this way, if there is an age trend related to the site, for example, it will be lost through the harmonization process, and the residualized measures will be incomplete or distorted. That is why a second harmonization model is proposed, this time called the "Adjusted linear regression model", meaning that we will "correct" the residualization or harmonization with care to preserve important variability due, for now, to age or sex in the measures. To do so, the covariables of interest are included as features in the regression model. Once the model was fitted, we removed only the site coefficient from the initial data, while age and sex trends were kept. Hence, the harmonization was adjusted on the covariates of interest. This second adjusted linear regression model can be written as follows:

$$X_i = \alpha_i + Z_{site}\beta_i + Z_{cov}\delta_i + \epsilon_i \tag{5}$$

where Z_{cov} contains the observations of the age and the sex (an $n \times 2$ matrix), δ_i is a 2×1 column vector of the age and sex coefficients of the regression, and the rest has the same notation as in Equation 1.

It can also be written for each subject, once again, to be closer to the literature's notations:

$$X_i k_j = \alpha_i + \gamma_{ik} + Z_{cov,j}\delta_i + \epsilon_i k_j \tag{6}$$

with the same notations as in Equation 2, where $Z_{cov,j}$ is the j-th line of the matrix Z_{cov}, corresponding to age and sex information of the subject j [2].

β_i and δ_i are estimated solving the OLS problem, and then the volumes are residualized or harmonized as follows:

$$\tilde{X}_i^{adj} = X_i - Z_{site}\hat{\beta}_i \tag{7}$$

or as follows:

$$\tilde{X}_{ik}^{adj} = X_{ikj} - \hat{\gamma}_{ik} \tag{8}$$

By removing only the site coefficient and keeping the term $Z_{cov}\hat{\delta}_i$, the biological information was preserved.

In this adjusted harmonization, where the site effect is still considered additive, the biological and site information can take forms other than the general ones proposed in the previous equations. In this way, we can draw inspiration from the work of Pomponio et al., who proposed an adaptation of the ComBat method called ComBat-GAM that we develop later, where they suggest considering the age as a quadratic term and not a linear term in the regression model [3]. By doing so, our model is not linear anymore but remains very close. The covariates of interest become the sex and the square of age, and they also add the intracranial volume (ICV), thus resulting in a generalized additive model (GAM). The site effect can also be modeled differently by adding information about the scanners used in the features. This is what Wachinger et al. did: they added as non-biological features (thus implying an inter-site variability that we wish to remove) the manufacturer of the scanner and the magnetic field strength, but they also thought that there was a non-explicit inter-site variability that was not captured by these parameters. Based on previous work in genome-wide association studies, they considered that this non-explicit variability can be captured by the principal components of the dataset, which they therefore add to the features responsible for the site effect [2].

After investigating two relatively similar residualization methods, we focus on a method called ComBat (for combining batches). According to the literature, this method presents several advantages compared to the first two harmonization methods that we explore further in the following after presenting the model. Like the two previous methods, the ComBat method considers the presence of an additive site effect in the harmonization model but goes further by considering the presence of a multiplicative site effect in the error term. It was Johnson and Li who introduced in 2007 how to deal with "batch effects" observed in gene expression microarrays [4]. In 2018, Fortin et al. used the same model to harmonize cortical thickness measurements (thickness of the human cerebral cortex) by MRI, which was closer to the type of measures we deal with in this study (brain images or ROIs). We write the model as follows:

$$X_i = \alpha_i + Z_{site}\beta_i + \psi_i\epsilon_i \qquad (9)$$

As previously, we find the additive term $Z_{site}\beta_i$, but now, we also have ψi, an $n \times n$ diagonal matrix, with a constant coefficient for patients from the same site corresponding to the multiplicative site effect for the ROI$_i$. α_i is still the average volume of the ROI$_i$, and ϵ_i is the $n \times 1$ error term that we assume to be normally distributed with an expected value of zero and variance σ^2. We also write the model at the subject scale as follows:

$$X_{ik_j} = \alpha_i + \gamma_{ik} + \psi_{ik}\epsilon_{ik_j} \qquad (10)$$

with the same notations as in Equation 2, where ψ_{ik} is the multiplicative effect of site k (the site of subject j) on ROI$_i$ [4].

ComBat, just like the previous model, can be adjusted on the biological covariables of interest. The idea of the adjustment is still to remove the site effect while preserving the age or sex information. We can write the adjusted model as follows:

$$X_i = \alpha_i + Z_{site}\,\beta_i + Z_{cov}\delta_i + \psi_i\epsilon_i \tag{11}$$

or at the subject scale as follows:

$$X_{ikj} = \alpha_i + \gamma_{ik} + Z_{cov,j}\delta_i + \psi_{ik}\epsilon_{ikj} \tag{12}$$

again with the same notations.

As before, we want to estimate the different parameters of the model and then remove the site parameters (γ_{ik} and ψ_{ik}). The main difference from the previous models, in addition to the introduction of a multiplicative site effect, is the estimation of the site parameters by the empirical Bayes method instead of the ordinary least squares estimation that was used for the first two models. According to the literature, using the empirical Bayes method is more robust, particularly for small sample sizes. This method assumes that the site often affects the features, or many of them, in the same way (higher variability, increased expression) and, therefore, that the site parameters share the same distributions across features (ROIs in our example). The information on all the features is thus used to estimate the parameters, which can be useful for small sample sizes, especially in managing outliers [5].

To do so, the estimation was implemented in two stages. The first one was a standardization of the data across features, which allowed the same magnitude of expression values for each region of interest (or any other type of feature). Using the notations of Equation 12, the standardized ROIs can be written as follows:

$$Z_{ikj} = \frac{\cdot X_{ikj}\cdots\hat{\alpha}_i\cdot -\cdot Z_{cov,j}\cdot\hat{\delta}_i}{\hat{\sigma}_i} \tag{13}$$

For standardization, the model parameter estimators $\hat{\alpha}_i$, $\hat{\delta}^i$, and $\hat{\gamma}_{ik}$ were determined by solving the ordinary least squares problem with a constraint $\sum_i n_i\hat{\gamma}_{ik} = 0$, where n_i is the number of subjects from site i, to make the parameters identifiable. As a reminder, σ^2_i is the variance of the error term ϵ_{ikj} and is estimated by

$$\widehat{\sigma_i^2} = \frac{1}{n}\sum_{kj}\left(X_{ikj} - \hat{\alpha}_i - \widehat{\gamma_{ik}} - Z_{cov,j}\hat{\delta}_i\right)^2$$

where n is the total number of patients.

After standardization, we estimate the additive and multiplicative site effect using the empirical Bayes method.

Once the estimators $\hat{\gamma}_{ik}{}^*$ and $\hat{\psi}_{ik}{}^*$ are calculated, the residualized data can be written as follows:

$$
\begin{aligned}
X_{ikj}^{comb,adj} &= \frac{\hat{\sigma}_i}{\hat{\psi}_{ik}^*}\left(Z_{ikj} - \hat{\gamma}_{ik}^*\right) + \alpha_i + Z_{cov,j}\hat{\delta}_i \\
&= \frac{X_{ikj} - \hat{\alpha}_i - Z_{cov,j}\hat{\delta}_i - \hat{\gamma}_{ik}^*}{\hat{\psi}_{ik}} + \hat{\alpha}_i + Z_{cov,j}\hat{\delta}_i
\end{aligned}
\tag{14}
$$

In this version, the harmonization was adjusted on the covariables of interest, but, as before, for the fixed effect models, we decided not to make adjustments at the risk of losing the important variability related to age or sex.

As previously, some extensions of this model were proposed by the literature. Wachinger et al. proposed including more information about the site in the ComBat model [2]. By being more precise in the site characteristics, non-biological variability can be better modeled and removed. In this way, in addition to the site origin of the patient, they also added the magnetic field strength of the scanner and the principal components of the dataset, as discussed for the fixed effect models. Their model can be written as follows:

$$X_i = \alpha_i + Z_{site}\beta_i + r\xi_i + Z_{cov}\delta_i + \psi_i\epsilon_i \tag{15}$$

with the same notations as previously, where r is an $n \times 4$ matrix containing the magnetic field strength, the two principal components of the dataset, and the scanner manufacturer for each patients; and ξ_i is the 4×1 parameter vector of the regression for the ROI_i or at the subject scale as follows:

$$\mathbf{X}_{ikj}\cdot = \cdot\alpha_i + \cdot\gamma_{ik} + \cdot\gamma_j\xi_i\cdot + \cdot Z_{cov,j}\delta_i\cdot + \cdot\Psi_{ik}\epsilon_{ikj} \tag{16}$$

where r_j is the j-th line of r, corresponding to the coefficients for patient j. The residualized data can be written as follows:

$$X_{ikj}^{comb,adj} = \frac{X_{ikj} - \hat{\alpha}_i - Z_{cov,j}\hat{\delta}_i - \widehat{\gamma}_{ik}^* - r_j\hat{\xi}_i^*}{\psi_{ik}} + \hat{\alpha}_i + Z_{cov,j}\hat{\delta}_i \qquad (17)$$

We separated Z_{site} and r to be close to Wachinger's notation. Wachinger et al. write their model like this to highlight their contribution, but we can group all non-biological variation under one notation to properly differentiate it from the covariates of interest that we want to preserve and thus gain clarity, which seems even better. In this way, we can keep the previous notations, Z_{site} and γ_{ik}, to include all the non-biological variables related to the site and thus keep the model written as in Equation 11 or 12.

In his work, Pomponio added a contribution to the ComBat model, calling his version the ComBat-GAM. He proposed not linearly modeling the variability related to biological covariates but rather capturing it through a generalized additive model, the theory of which was briefly noted in the previous section. The model can be written as follows:

$$X_{ikj} \cdots = \alpha_i \ldots + \gamma_{ik} \cdots + f_i(Z_{cov}, j) + \psi_{ik}\epsilon_{ikj} \qquad (18)$$

with the same notations as in Equation 16, where f_i is a smooth function allowing nonlinear age trends in the model [3]. Note that they also added the ICV mentioned earlier in the biological covariates of interest as an additional contribution to Johnson's version. This showed that any relevant biological information that may explain a part of the dataset variability must be included in the model to better discriminate non-biological variability related to the site. Otherwise, some of this biological variability may be captured by the site coefficient and then inappropriately removed. Similarly, the more site information we bring into the model, the more accurate we will be at estimating inter-site variability. We were able to explore three methods of harmonization for the data, allowing them to be cleaned from the site effect. Few results from the literature show that the ComBat method performs well, even better than fixed effect methods for small sample sizes.

5.3 PROPOSED METHODOLOGY

As explained previously, the second and the third residualization methods adjusted the harmonization on the covariates of interest, which we usually want to predict after residualization to evaluate the models. Indeed, the goal of harmonizing brain data is to be able to conduct reliable studies allowing us to understand certain human behaviors, to anticipate the diagnosis of certain neurological diseases such as schizophrenia or epilepsy, or to predict the effectiveness of a treatment, and this is why we need methods preserving the biological variability of data. One way to ensure this is to try to predict the covariates of interest to assess this preservation, as seen in the literature results. However, when the harmonization method used was adjusted on a covariate of interest that we wish to predict later, we were faced with a bias when predicting the latter. This cannot occur with harmonization by a simple linear regression model, since we do not adjust on any covariate, but can be a problem when adjusting the linear regression model or ComBat model on age, for example. That is why the harmonization model for predicting age or any other covariables used in the adjustment must be fitted on a different dataset than the one used to evaluate it. The methodology used in the literature does not seem to pay attention to this detail, which could alter the quality of the results to a greater or lesser extent. The method adopted is shown in Figure 5.1.

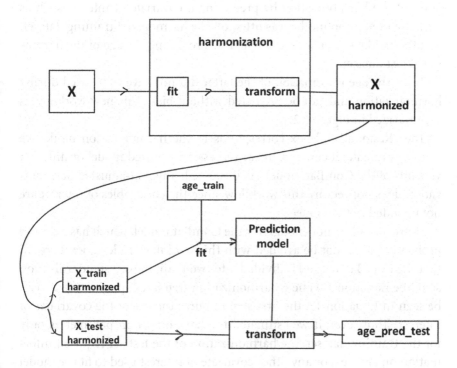

FIGURE 5.1   Literature workflow for model evaluation.

That is, the harmonization model is estimated on the whole dataset, which is then harmonized, and then the model is evaluated by adopting a classical cross-validation scheme to predict age, for example, as Fortin et al. did [6].

This scheme starts after harmonization, which means that the test data on which we want to predict age have already been adjusted during harmonization using the information on age and other covariables of interest, which is the origin of the bias. This is confirmed by the structure of the ComBat code used by Fortin et al., which does not allow separating the fit from the transform at all, but also by the one used by Wachinger et al., which is just an adaptation of the original version (ComBat++ [2]).

For the adjusted linear regression model, the solution to remove the bias mentioned previously is rather simple. The dataset must be separated into training and test datasets before estimating the harmonization model. Parameters γ_{ik} and δ_i of the model (see Equation 6) are then estimated using only the training dataset. We next harmonized the whole dataset using these parameters, as in Equation 8. We then proceeded to the evaluation of the harmonization by predicting a covariate of interest such as age. The prediction model was fitted on the harmonized training dataset, and the model scores were evaluated by predicting the age of the harmonized test dataset.

Thus, the age information of the latter did not have to be used during harmonization and can be predicted without bias. This new workflow is summarized in Figure 5.2.

The "Residualizer" box corresponds to the harmonization model we want to evaluate; it can be a linear regression adjusted model or different versions of the ComBat model. As discussed, any non-adjusted harmonization does not require this workflow since the covariables of interest are not included in the model.

However, this is not enough for the ComBat model, which has a deeper problem that cannot be avoided with this workflow. Indeed, let us recall that the ComBat method is divided into two main steps: a standardization step (see Equation 13) and a harmonization step (see Equation 14). As can be seen in Equation 13, the first step requires the use of the covariates of interest. Thus, even if we estimated the harmonization parameters only for the training dataset, the harmonization of the test set required information on age, sex, or any other covariate of interest used to fit the model

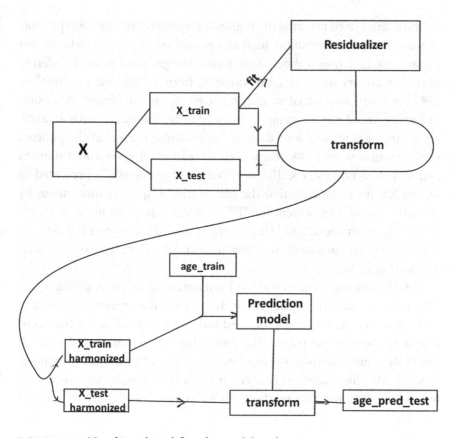

FIGURE 5.2   Non-biased workflow for model evaluation.

(principal components (PCs), ICV). It then becomes irrelevant to predict a covariate of interest of the test, set such as age, after harmonization to evaluate the harmonization model. We still did it, by reducing the bias by adopting the model evaluation scheme, and compared the results to the literature. In keeping with the way of avoiding bias and also to avoid any variability related to the diagnosis since it is not problematic at this stage, we used only control patients for now. To test our methods, we first had access to a dataset with average gray matter volumes for 280 regions of interest in the brain for just under 7000 patients at 24 different sites. Grey matter volumes are measured by magnetic resonance techniques. Working on the regions of interest allowed us to reduce the data size in terms of number of features.

The dataset used presents the regions of interest of nearly 7000 patients as well as other information such as age and sex of the subjects. In our dataset, we had nine cohorts that group images from several different sites. The cohort size was quite variable, from 65 subjects for "npc" to 2897 for "corr". Recall that we only had control patients. There are 24 sites in Europe and America, ranging from 10 to 1639 subjects, with an average of 287 patients and a median of 142 patients. The age of the patients varied from 6 years to 88 years, with a mean of 28 years and 4 months and a median of 23 years. The distribution of sex by site is presented in Figure 5.3. It can be seen that the distribution is quite homogeneous by site and around 50%, except for "NKI", which has 100% males but contains only 10 subjects, and "Utah", which has 100% females but only 62 subjects. The whole dataset was 52% men and 48% women, so the distribution is quite fair.

This dataset was used to test the harmonization methods discussed in the previous sections. For harmonization by the linear regression model, each region of interest was processed independently, while for harmonization by the ComBat model, the processing was common and used all the ROIs simultaneously. We also tested them on "handmade" toy datasets. We also had access to the patients' brain images, so we could have tested the harmonization methods on the voxels, but we have focused on the ROIs.

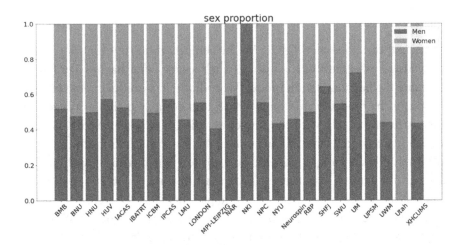

FIGURE 5.3   Sex proportion across sites.

5.4 RESULTS AND DISCUSSION

We tested different aspects of the harmonization methods. First, their ability to remove the site effect from the data. Second, their ability to preserve the variability linked to the covariates of interest such as age or sex as mentioned in the state of the art. Finally, we will discuss some possible improvements.

5.4.1 Site Prediction

The first point to check is the effectiveness of the harmonization, that is, whether the undesirable site effect has been removed. To do this, we predict the site effect using the logistic regression model and the workflow detailed in the previous section. We expect a significant reduction in site prediction scores after harmonization. There are 24 sites, so the chance level is $1/24 = 0.042$. To split the dataset, we used the StratifiedKFold function of scikit learn, allowing an equivalent representation of the sites in each fold. This avoided under-represented sites or sites not represented at all in one of the loops of the cross-validation. We prevented the distortion of the results. We performed a five-fold stratified cross-validation with $C = 0.1$ as the tuning parameter for the logistic regression model. We were not necessarily looking for the best parameter, but we wanted to fix it for all the methods so that the comparison of the scores would be relevant. We also used a L2-penalty for the same reasons as the ridge regression model.

The results are presented in Figure 5.4. The first line ("Raw") corresponds to the score on the site prediction before harmonization. Looking at the balanced accuracy of 0.814, we see a very good ability to predict the site of origin of the data before processing. This high score was our reference to show the presence of site-related variability in the data. The second row shows the prediction results after harmonization by the unadjusted

Harmonization method	Balanced accuracy
Raw	0.814 ±0.0097
Linear regression non-adjusted	0.042 ±0.000
Linear regression adjusted	0.090 ±0.0028
ComBat	0.0580 ±0.0018
ComBat_sklearn	0.0904 ±0.0030

FIGURE 5.4 Evaluation of harmonization methods by site prediction.

linear regression model (see Equations 2 and 3). We can see that the balanced accuracy dropped drastically and reached the chance level of 1/24, showing that the site effect was removed. The scores after harmonization by the adjusted linear regression model (see Equations 6 and 7) are presented in line 3. The balanced accuracy was 0.90, which was slightly above the chance level and the previous method but well below the initial performance, showing that the inter-site variability was well removed. This method performed slightly worse than the previous method. This was due to the fact that the adjustment on the covariates of interest reintroduced information on the site in the case of correlation.

In any case, this method removed the site effect satisfactorily, and if it also preserved the biological variability at the cost of a slight deterioration of the harmonization, it meets the need successfully. Hence, we have the results of two versions of the ComBat model. The first one is the one used in the literature, where the harmonization parameters were estimated on the whole dataset, which introduced a bias, as explained previously. The second version (ComBat sklearn) is the version adapted to the new workflow, allowing us to reduce but still not avoid this bias. The values of the balanced accuracy showed that both versions allowed removal of the inter-site variability since they are much lower than our reference. We also note that the biased version led to a lower score than the unbiased version. Finally, the unbiased version performed as well as the adjusted linear regression model, which confirmed the effectiveness of the ComBat method. In summary, we were able to successfully verify the presence of inter-site variability via the very good prediction of the site before harmonization, and we also found that the three harmonization methods allowed us to remove the inter-site variability correctly. We now turn to the preservation of biological variability.

5.4.2 Sex Prediction

To see if the information on the sex of the patient has not been lost during the harmonization, we carried out the same reasoning. We predicted the covariate of interest using the same scheme (see Figure 5.2 before and after harmonization) and then discuss the results. We again performed a five-fold stratified cross validation with $C = 0.1$ as tuning parameter for the logistic regression model. The prediction scores are presented in Figure 5.5. The first row still shows the prediction results before harmonization. This time we looked at the balanced accuracy, the area under curve, and the sensitivity. The balanced accuracy of 0.788 as well as the AUC of 0.867 and

Harmonization method	Balanced accuracy	AUC	Sensitivity
Raw	0.788 ±0.010	0.867 ±0.008	0.872 ±0.003
Linear regression non-adjusted	0.858 ±0.005	0.930 ±0.003	0.874 ±0.004
Linear regression adjusted	**0.871 ±0.005**	0.937 ±0.002	0.887 ±0.005
ComBat	0.8810 ±0.0065	0.931 ±0.004	0.872 ±0.006
ComBat sklearn	0.8812 ±0.0069	0.931 ±0.004	0.872 ±0.006

FIGURE 5.5　Evaluation of harmonization methods by sex prediction.

the sensitivity of 0.872 demonstrated that we managed to predict the sex very accurately before harmonization.

After using different harmonization methods, we noticed an improvement in the sex prediction scores. This showed that the variability linked to sex was not lost during the harmonization whether it was linear (adjusted or not) or by ComBat model. We even noticed a slight improvement in the prediction scores, which meets our criteria successfully. Indeed, the preservation of the biological variability must be translated beyond the stability of the prediction efficiency by an improvement of the latter since the non-biological variability that is detrimental to the quality of the data was removed. This is what we observed here, even if it remains slight. The change in prediction scores between the raw data and the harmonized data is small since there is a weak correlation between site and sex, as can be seen in Figure 5.3, so harmonizing does not impact sex-related variability. We therefore next looked at how age was impacted. Before looking at how age was impacted, we noticed a few more points. The first one is the improvement of the prediction scores between the linear regression model and the adjusted linear regression model, which shows the interest of introducing the biological covariates to be preserved in the model. The second point is the fact that the ComBat method had the best results and that there is no difference between the initial version and the version calculating the harmonization parameters on the training dataset only. This is surely due to the methodological bias already discussed for age, that is, the fact that the standardization across features of the ComBat model requires information on the covariates of interest that we try to predict next. Second, the fact that both versions of the ComBat model resulted in the same scores shows that the introduced workflow does not remove the bias for the ComBat model, or at least not completely. The interest remains present and justified for the adjusted linear regression model where it allows us to avoid any bias. The results are moreover slightly lower than when we simply estimated the harmonization parameters on the whole dataset and when the cross-validation loop was only introduced from the prediction of the covariates of interest.

5.4.3 Age Prediction

Still from the same perspective, let's look at the prediction of age, which is another biological covariate of interest. As a reminder, robust prediction of the biological covariates of interest will provide confidence in the subsequent prediction of treatment efficacy or disease occurrence. So it is important to make sure that the harmonized data still allow for their correct prediction, or, in other words, that the biological variability has been preserved through harmonization.

The age prediction results are shown in Figure 5.6. Once again, we adopted the same evaluation scheme (see Figure 5.2). The age was predicted by the ridge regression, with an L2 penalty, by fixing the tuning parameter for all harmonizations.

The first line shows again the age prediction results from the raw data. We looked each time at the R-squared (R^2) and the mean absolute error (MAE). The R-squared value of 0.811 and the MAE of 4.994 show that age can be predicted very well from the raw data, indicating the presence of age-related variability in the data. Note that the prediction scores after harmonization by the unadjusted linear regression model (R^2 of 0.291 and a MAE of 9.610) are very poor, showing that age-related variability has been removed, along with undesirable site-related variability, which is exactly what we wished to avoid during harmonization and again testifies to the importance of adjusting models on the covariates of interest. This is in fact the case for the results presented in the last three rows, and we see a clear improvement in the prediction scores for both versions of the ComBat (biased and unbiased) model and for the adjusted linear regression model. The prediction scores are slightly higher than the raw data, which means

Harmonization method	r2 ±SE	Mean absolute error ±SE
Raw	0.811 ±0.003	4.994 ±0.054
Linear regression non-adjusted	0.291 ±0.013	9.610 ±0.082
Linear regression adjusted	0.823 ±0.003	4.821 ±0.050
ComBat	0.8361 ±0.0032	4.6997 ±0.0625
neuroComBat_sklearn	0.8267 ±0.0049	4.7412 ±0.0744

FIGURE 5.6 Evaluation of harmonization methods by age prediction.

not only that these three methods preserved the age-related variability but also that removing non-biological site-related variability allows for slightly better prediction of the biological covariates even if the increase is not clear (the lack of improvement may be related to the type of data and will be discussed again in the following). Note also that the adjusted linear regression model and the unbiased version of the ComBat (neuro-ComBat sklearn) model scores were slightly lower than the initial ComBat model. This indicates the presence of bias in the evaluation of the initial ComBat model and also the ability of our evaluation scheme to remove some of this bias (since ComBat sklearn performs worse), although, again, normalization across the ComBat model features requires information about the covariates of interest that we are trying to predict next, which means that the bias cannot be fully removed by this scheme. Nevertheless, it does allow for the adjusted regression model, and we see that the scores of the latter and neuroComBat sklearn model are very close, which makes the biased version of the ComBat model a very good candidate despite a slightly biased evaluation.

5.4.4 Discussion

As explained before, it is not really rigorous to predict age or sex to evaluate the ComBat model since they are part of the covariables of interest that we try to preserve. But we did see the impact of the harmonization on age and did look at the life-span trajectory as presented by Johnson et al. in Figure 5.7 [4].

In red, we have the patients from the EMBARC study, and those in green are from the VDLC study, each study containing several sites. We can observe a high variability in the data from EMBARC in the raw data compared to the green points. We note that this inter-site variability is largely reduced by the ComBat harmonization, which is an indication of efficiency. The common trajectory of the two studies is preserved during the harmonization. Furthermore, the correlation between the median of the cortical thickness was calculated. It is −0.70 before harmonization and −0.79 after harmonization by the ComBat model, showing that the inter-site variability was removed while preserving that related to age. This could be evaluated without bias and confirms what was observed with the age-biased prediction. We can also observe from the same part of the article that the removal of the site effect without adjustment is thus again fatal to the preservation of the biological variability. We can similarly evaluate harmonization by

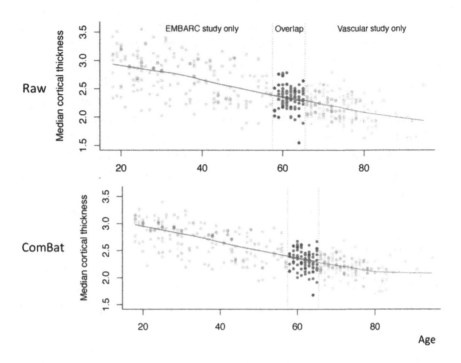

FIGURE 5.7   Life-span trajectory before and after harmonization with ComBat [6].

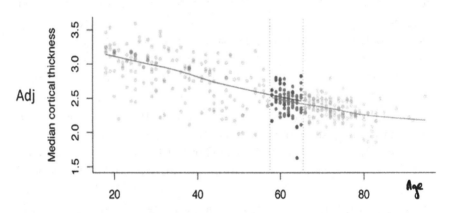

FIGURE 5.8   Life-span trajectory after adjusted linear residualization [6].

the adjusted linear regression model, even though it could be evaluated in the previous sections without bias.

In Figure 5.8, we can see that the high variability in the EMBARC data (red) was reduced and the common trajectory was preserved.

The correlation between the median cortical thickness and age was −0.77 after this harmonization, which is almost as good as the ComBat method. These two points show the effectiveness of this harmonization. The latter and ComBat method performed equally well on these large datasets.

5.5 CONCLUSION

We conclude that the prediction of the covariates of interest as presented in the literature presents a bias that we have tried to limit (for the ComBat method) or even remove (for the linear regression model) by introducing an evaluation scheme that does not estimate the coefficients of the harmonization on the whole dataset. At the same time, the methods in the literature were adapted to the new workflow (see Figures 5.1 and 5.2). We tested the new workflow on a dataset, including the regions of interest of 7000 patients, and we were able to successfully confirm the good performances presented in the literature, thus showing that, although visible, the bias did not have a huge impact on the evaluation of the models. But this bias poses a fundamental problem for the ComBat method, which necessarily uses the information of the covariates of interest during harmonization (more precisely in the standardization step), which are often target data, especially for post-harmonization predictions. There is thus a non-conforming use of the ComBat method with the basic principles of machine learning, where the target information of the test set that one wishes to predict must never be introduced beforehand.

We also explored other ways to evaluate the harmonizations without bias, in particular by looking at the life-span trajectory, allowing us to see the impact of the site effect and the harmonizations on the variability of the data and on the general trend of the data along the life span of the patients. In this context, the ComBat method can be used, but generally, one will need to work on the protected variables after harmonization, so the use of this method seems limited.

ACKNOWLEDGMENTS

The data used are from open access cohorts. The data distribution is detailed in Figure 5.9.

Study	Control patient
corr	2897
gsp	1639
icbm	977
localizer	82
ixi	559
mpi-leipzig	317
nar	323
npc	65
rbp	40
	6899

FIGURE 5.9 Cohorts.

REFERENCES

1. C. Wachinger, A. Rieckmann, and S. Pölsterl, "Detect and correct bias in multi-site neuroimaging datasets," Medical Image Analysis, vol. 67, Jan. 2021.
2. G. Zhu, B. Jiang, L. Tong, Y. Xie, G. Zaharchuk, and M. Wintermark, "Applications of deep learning to neuro-imaging techniques," English, Frontiers in Neurology, vol. 10, 2019.
3. Qshick, Ridge Regression for Better Usage, Towards Data Science, Jan 2019. [Online]. https://towardsdatascience.com/ridge-regression-for-better-usage-2f19b3a202db (visited on 07/09/2023).
4. J. Lakkis, D. Wang, Y. Zhang, G. Hu, K. Wang, H. Pan, L. Ungar, M. P. Reilly, X. Li, and M. Li, "A joint deep learning model for simultaneous batch effect correction, denoising and clustering in single-cell transcriptomics," en, bioRxiv, p. 310003, Sep. 2020.13.
5. Frédéric Joliot Institute for Life Sciences—Welcome. [Online]. https://joliot.cea.fr/drf/joliot/en (visited on 08/31/2021).
6. J.-P. Fortin, D. Parker, B. Tunc̨, T. Watanabe, M. A. Elliott, K. Ruparel, D. R. Roalf, T. D. Satterthwaite, R. C. Gur, R. E. Gur, R. T. Schultz, R. Verma, and R. T. Shinohara, "Harmonization of multi-site diffusion tensor imaging data," NeuroImage, vol. 161, pp. 149–170, Nov. 2017.

CHAPTER 6

Feature-Ranking Methods for RNA Sequencing Data

Girija Rani Karetla, Quang Vinh Nguyen,
Simeon J. Simoff, Daniel R. Catchpoole,
and Paul J. Kennedy

6.1 INTRODUCTION

Viruses, pathogens, fungi, bacteria, and other infectious organisms are all around us. Human bodies, for the most part, have a basic defence system against illnesses caused by these substances. In the modern environment, the rise of superbugs and the resurgence of diseases including influenza, Zika, and Ebola are major concerns. Further research into these illnesses and disorders is critical [1]. With the development of cheaper high-throughput technologies, research progress and experiments on sequencing analysis have grown dramatically. This has led to the creation of huge, heterogeneous datasets at lower costs for experimental analysis.

Recent advances in sequencing technology, like next generation sequencing (NGS) via ribonucleic acid sequencing (RNA-Seq), have made it possible to measure the levels of expression of many transcripts at the same time [2]. Using this information, several undefined methods based on expression levels have been developed. Classification is currently considered a useful method for cancer identification and diagnosis as well as the discovery of possible biomarkers for diseases [3]. Exogenous RNA substances (viruses) can also be identified using this approach for RNA-Seq data. By using machine learning (ML) approaches and classification algorithms, these traits can now be easily found in RNA-Seq data.

DOI: 10.1201/9781003292357-6

In the last few decades, classification has been used a lot more because it helps find biomarkers for cancer and sets therapeutic goals [4]. RNA-Seq data can be used to find disease-related genes by putting them into many different groups based on their properties. Many different computational methods have been developed to do this. However, these methods and technologies for studying large datasets are still limited. In addition, there is a limited possibility of classifying and analyzing RNA-Seq data, which makes it much harder to assign the cancer samples into appropriate groups [5].

Dimensionality reduction is a hard problem to solve when there are a lot of features or attributes to think about. Some examples of these areas are "feature extraction and text categorisation in digital documents, gene expression microarray analysis, and molecule segmentation in bioinformatics and combinatorial challenges" [5]. In such a scenario, it is practical to demand that you narrow down the available characteristics to a manageable group in order to extract the relevant data. Important in this context is a preprocessing operation known as "feature ranking" which ranks a set of features according to how well they identify a target value [6]. Similar to other supervised learning algorithms, the features are ordered based on an input training set. Using feature-ranking algorithms as a classification method, these kinds of things can be added to decision trees. These algorithms can also be used to create a filter for feature selection. One way to get data ready for analysis by data mining methods like classification and clustering is to choose features. After removing duplicates and other junk from a dataset, feature selection pulls out a subset of the initial characteristics [6].

This chapter compares the different ways of ranking features, such as statistical ranking, machine learning-based ranking, and deep learning-based ranking, for RNA-Seq and gene expression data. The method under discussion considers both how well feature-ranking techniques can predict the future and how input variables interact with one another. The input features are ranked using three different methods: a statistical technique based on statistics; a machine learning-based method called support vector machine (SVM); and a deep learning-based method called deep neural network (DNN), with the calculated standard errors acting as a key variable. Each of these methods evaluates the importance of a variable on its own based on the assumptions it makes about the regression function connecting the predictors and the predicted variable. Each dataset will be divided into two categories, each of which will be used in a different context for training and testing the model's performance. Based on a defined reduction threshold, the lowest-ranking characteristics are removed from each group. Empirical findings were compared with the existing dataset and various feature selection strategies on a wide range of real datasets. The findings show that feature selection increases classification accuracy in principle, and integrating features using various heterogeneous feature-ranking algorithms provides a more robust feature set. Compared to other feature selection methods, our study shows that the deep learning-based feature selection method outperforms other methods at predicting outcomes.

6.2 RELATED WORKS

Deep learning techniques for cancer detection and significant gene detection for breast cancer analysis are discussed in detail. A stacked denoising auto-encoder is used to extract meaningful features from gene expression contours [7, 8]. To identify if the extra features are effective in the cancer detection process, supervised classification models are employed to evaluate the recovered representation's performance. Also, stacked auto-encoder connection matrices are utilised to find a collection of highly interacting genes [8]. The highly interacting genes might be potential cancer biomarkers, such as for breast cancer screening. Jabeen, Ahmad, and Raza provide a comprehensive discussion on ML techniques for RNA-Seq data classification and their application [1]. Together, these advances in bioinformatics and ML-based categorisation can lead to effective toolboxes for classifying transcriptome RNA-Seq data into suitable categories.

An efficient deep gene selection (DGS) algorithm for choosing related genes that are quite complex for the sample classes is provided [9]. It has the potential to minimise the number of genes in microarray datasets. Experiments on the comparison of DGS with other typical and advanced gene-choice processes reveal that the DGS method outperforms others for significant gene selection, classification accuracy, and processing cost [9]. Schaack used gene expression data to investigate the molecular-level sample categorisation of sepsis. The differential expression result is compared with ML techniques, including random forest, decision tree, deep learning neural networks, and support vector machine [10]. The expression data are progressively decreased at multiple levels to assess diagnostic robustness. Clustering expression data based on differential expression genes enable the partial identification of sepsis samples. This study shows that the deep learning network method is the most stable method because deleting differentially expressed genes has almost no effect on them [11].

The gene encoder is a model for classifying cancer samples that chooses features without any help from a person. Several filter methods are aggregated in the initial stage of this work. The process can analyse principal components, relationships, and feature selections based on spectral data. A genetic algorithm is then applied, which uses auto-encoder-based clustering to analyse the chromosome. For classification purposes, the resultant feature subsets are used. In this process, support vector machine, random forest, and K-nearest neighbour are used to avoid having to rely on just one classifier. Using clustering, tests are used to evaluate certain features, change the best parameters, and choose the best classifiers [12].

6.3 RNA-SEQUENCING AND ITS WORKFLOW

It has been found that RNA-Seq is a good transcriptome sequencing NGS method for getting a full picture of the RNA transcripts in test samples. RNA-Seq is a method that looks at how many transcripts are being transcribed at the same time [13]. The main way RNA-Seq is used to study disease is to do an expression analysis on the original sequence data of the disease after it has been normalised, then build a specific network framework for identifying genes and evaluating their overall network properties [14]. Multiple genes linked to the disease could be identified using this molecular biological technique. These recently discovered genes might be used as strategies for therapeutic development. Figure 6.1 illustrates the RNA-Seq analysis technique's sequential phases [15].

Differential expression analysis is used to classify the main cancer-metabolism–related hub genes in more detail. A gene or other regions of interest could be detected using this method [16]. From a computational perspective, [17] provides a simplified machine learning process for data classification. When interacting with RNA-Seq data, a similar technique that is shown in Figure 6.2 may be utilised for classifying RNA sequencing data.

6.3.1 Challenges in High-Dimensional RNA-Seq Data

Rapid improvements in sequencing technology have led to a huge increase in the amount of relevant sequencing data, which is used to make important scientific discoveries in biology and medicine. Most individual transcriptome RNA-Seq datasets keep getting bigger, which makes it harder to

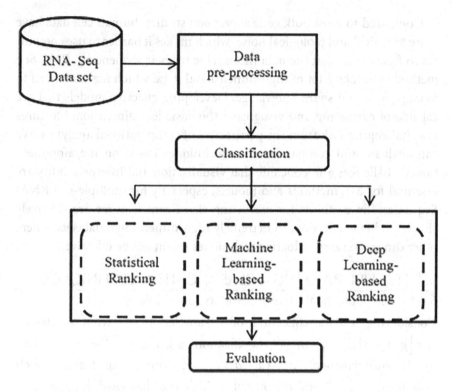

FIGURE 6.1 RNA-Seq data analysis.

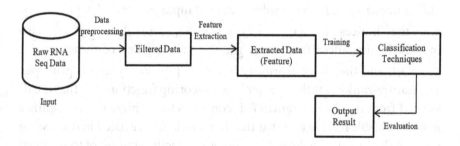

FIGURE 6.2 Classification workflow.

analyse them because they have so many dimensions. This new generation of sequencing technology focuses on the sequence data from human cells, which can reveal a lot about how complex biological systems work. Due to the large number of cells in the samples, it goes without saying that data from human cells are hard to process on a computer.

Compared to most bulk gene expression studies, human cell data have more technical and biological noise, which makes it harder to use computers to figure out what the data mean. Due to their sequencing, RNA-Seq methods produce a lot of high-dimensional data, which makes it hard to manage data and share knowledge. Developing effective models that are capable of extracting and visualising the basic low-dimensional features is a challenging task from the perspective of computational analytics. We can evaluate and compare various techniques based on the aforementioned challenges and conclude that visualisation and interpretability are essential for ML methods and models, especially for multiple-cell RNA-Seq data. The methods for extracting significant features are relatively simple and efficient, even in extremely high-dimensional datasets, where other dimensionality reduction techniques might not be effective.

6.4 FEATURE RANKING—CLASSIFICATION TECHNIQUES

6.4.1 Using Statistical Measures for Feature Ranking

Considering a data collection of z samples $F = [1]$ from u classes, $G = \{g_p : p = 1, \ldots, u\}$ in a classification algorithm. The input vector is v-dimensional, $a_t = \{a_{tq} : q = 1, \ldots, v\}$, containing feature labels $H = \{h_q : q = 1, \ldots v\}$, and the output variable is a class label, $b_t \{g_1, \ldots, g_u\}$, for the tth instance. Each input variable a_{tq} is re-sampled to the unit interval [0, 1] to use a linear transformation that maintains the dataset's distribution unchanged. Let's consider the set of input matrices $A = \{a_1, \ldots, a_z\}$, and the indices $Q = \{1, \ldots, z\}. Q_p = \{t : t = 1, \ldots, z \text{ and } b_t = g_p$ are also indexes for instances from class g_p. The primary key of these cases is $z_p = |Q_p|$, and they have a priority based on probability L_p. In principle, any feature-ranking technique includes a scoring function R (.) that is calculated from the data instances F. It considers that a higher score signifies a more valuable feature and that the characteristics are listed in decreasing order of their values by default. It employs a specific amount of top-ranked characteristics in its experiments to utilise feature ranking for generating predictors. Consider $A' = a_1, \ldots, a_z$ obtained from the matrix set A, using a feature selection procedure, where $a_{t'}$ is a v'-dimensional vector and $v' < v$. Similarly, by eliminating $v - v'$ features from vectors a_t in A', A' is produced. The following is a definition of a ranking criterion:

$$P(A') = \frac{1}{2} \sum_{q=1}^{u} L_q \frac{1}{z_q} \sum_{p=1}^{u} L_p \frac{1}{z_q} \sum_{t \in Q_q} \sum_{w \in Q_p} f(a_t, a_{w'}) \tag{1}$$

where $f(a_t, a_w)$ denotes a distance metric, which is commonly the Euclidean norm. L_p, the class probability density, can be calculated as $\frac{z_p}{z}$ for class g_p.

That is, the unit interval [0, 1] is split into ten equal measures, and the frequency of instances in every part is measured. The class density function h_p is used to represent the histogram of samples from class g_p in each feature. These class density curves are shown in Figure 6.1 for the first feature of the Iris dataset [18], where the samples of each class are randomly distributed in discrete vertical segments.

After standardising the class probability densities acquired for that feature, $s_q (q = 1, \ldots, v)$, StatFR calculates the score value $E(q, p) = E(s_q, g_p)$ for all classes $g_p (p = 1, \ldots, u)$. $E(q, p)$ is a scoring function that may be used to calculate probabilities to determine the class. The between-class distance, F_p, the inter-class overlapping measure C_p, and the estimation of class impurity h_p are all calculated using different variations of the class density function for g_p. Each of these indicators appears to have certain differentiating power on its own, but their contribution to the scoring function should be more efficient. Although the weighted sum of these measures (i.e. $E(s_q, g_p) = w_1 F_p + w_2 C_p + w_3 H_p$) is more prevalent in tri-objective optimisation methods, assigning or learning the required weights is frequently a difficult task. The research in this reference aims at certain predefined unique weights.

Nevertheless, in this study, the metrics are multiplied to highlight their effective proportion to the scoring system. Furthermore, a low value against two various rates of F_p, C_p, or H_p will significantly lower the score in Equation 2, although in the instance of weighted sum, this minimum value may be ignored completely. As a result, the scoring system is defined as follows:

$$E(s_q, g_p) = F_p \times C_p \times H_p \qquad (2)$$

For class g_p, F_p, C_p, and H_p are generated, provided the feature S_q is analyzed.

The first measure, F_p, computes the distance between each target and its non-target classes using the performance metrics. Given the fact that StatFR uses this measure in their scoring systems, there are significant difference. First, StatFR uses a different concept of non-target class. Then, they utilise two distinct techniques for determining the mean and standard deviation of samples in every class.

$$\alpha_p = \frac{1}{z_p} \sum_{t \in Q_p} a_{tq} \tag{3}$$

and

$$\gamma_p^2 = \frac{1}{z_p} \sum_{t \in Q_p} \left(a_{tq} - \alpha_p \right)^2 \tag{4}$$

StatFR, on the other hand, applies the probability density h_j class for this. As a result, the mean of class C_j may be calculated as:

$$\alpha_p = \frac{\int_l h_{p'} f_l}{\int_l h_p f_l} = \frac{\sum_{t \in Q_p} h_p \left(a_{tq} \right) \times a_{tq}}{\sum_{t \in Q_p} h_p a_{tq}} \tag{5}$$

The significance of feature s_q is represented by L. If the normalised value of the class density function h_q is regarded as the fuzzy membership function, this derivation of the mean is equivalent to the centroid of the region defuzzification approach in the Mamdani fuzzy inference system. Class g_p 's variance may be calculated the same way:

$$\gamma_p^2 = \frac{\int_l h_{p'} f_l}{\int_l h_p f_l} - \left(\alpha_p \right)^2 \tag{6}$$

The between-class distance is defined as follows using these classifications:

$$F_p = \frac{\left(\alpha_p - \bar{\alpha}_p \right)^2}{\gamma_p^2 + \bar{\gamma}_p^2} \tag{7}$$

where $\bar{\alpha}_p$ and $\bar{\gamma}_p$ are membership of the non-target class.

F_p evaluates the distance between the centroid of target and non-target groups, ignoring the overlaps among them, which are also highlighted as disadvantages of Fisher's criterion. *StatFR* specifies the inter-class overlapping metric as follows to combine this component in the scoring function:

$$C_p = 1 - \frac{\widetilde{x}_p}{\widehat{x}_p} \tag{8}$$

where $\widetilde{x}_p$ and $\widehat{x}_p$ represent the area under the curve of the class density functions $\widetilde{h}_p$ and $\widehat{h}_p$, respectively. In other words,

$$\widehat{x}_p = \int_l \widehat{h}_p f_l \tag{9}$$

$$\widehat{h}_p = h_p \vee \overline{h}_p = min\left(h_p \overline{h}_p\right) \tag{10}$$

$$\widetilde{h}_p = h_p \wedge \overline{h}_p = min\left(h_p \overline{h}_p\right) \tag{11}$$

$$h_p = \frac{x_p}{\left(x_p + \overline{x}_p\right)} \tag{12}$$

6.4.2 Random Forest

The ensemble approach also includes a random forest (RF). It's a collection of many classification and regression trees (CARTs) that have not been used yet. Predictions from numerous weak forest classifier trees are averaged in RF to form a coherent classifier that gives the highest accurate prediction result [1, 19]. First, individual tree training sets are established by bootstrapping the original sample data. Following that, each of the decision trees is bagged after being trained on this bootstrapped sample dataset. Then, to develop the tree, RF selects various features to divide at each node [20]. Other statistical and machine learning algorithms, such as an SVM, are less flexible and have fewer customisable parameters. Allow a random vector to be created for the tth tree. As stated in Equation 13, it is unchanged by preceding random vectors with the same distribution.

$$\beta_t \ldots \ldots \beta_{t+1} \tag{13}$$

A tree may be constructed using the training dataset to produce a classifier $h\ (a, \beta_t)$, where a is an input vector. A random vector β_v is formed using counts provided by the V training set during the bagging phase. As illustrated in Eq. 14, a random forest is an ensemble classifier composed of many tree-structured classifiers.

$$\left\{h(a, \beta_t), t = 1, \ldots\right\} \tag{14}$$

Each β_t independent random vector and tree contribute to selecting the optimal effective form at input a. Without changing the training set, RFs are more effective than boosting and adaptive bagging. They have high precision and help to eliminate discrimination.

After the technique has formed enough trees, the most relevant class for prediction must be identified [21]. A bootstrap resampling procedure is used in an RF to divide a random feature. A subset of characteristics is defined for analysis at each tree node before training. Because bootstrapping is a sampling method based on repetitive substitution of training data, certain sequences may be ignored or duplicated in the sample. An out-of-bag (OOB) sample would be used to replace the missing sequences. Typically, about two-thirds of the training sequences are used to build a forest, and the other one-third is ignored as OOB. The OOB sequences could be utilised to anticipate efficiency because they are not committed to the forest formation process. The forest is constructed using the second third of the training sequences [19]. The average error of one-third of the OOB training data points is identified. As a result of the bootstrap resampling procedure, the OOB part is used to do simultaneous cross-validation, provided OOB error rates as a significant performance metric for the random forest method for prediction [21].

The results of each feature are then transferred among the remaining two-thirds of the training data, and the OOB error is determined using the newly trained data once more. To overcome the dimensionality curse, the RF technique can also be used to prioritise the relevance of these traits based on a subset of them. Only the most important aspects are then investigated further [22]. The modelling biases of a dataset or feature could be substantially decreased by splitting features. In this stage, each of the randomly chosen characteristics is subjected to either a non-parametric or a parametric technique to construct a decision tree. As a result, users have a collection of multiple decision trees in the form of an RF with more classification functionality and unbiased feature analysis [22].

6.4.3 Deep Stacking Network

The weight parameter, which includes the input network weight matrices I and the output network weight matrices O in each component, is learned from the training dataset using a basic tuning and learning method. Over the whole v number of training samples, let $A = \left[a_1, \ldots, a_q, \ldots, a_v \right]$ be the training vectors and $U = \left[u_1, \ldots, u_q, \ldots, u_v \right]$ be the target vectors.

Equation 15 shows the result of this deep stacking network (DSN) learning system:

$$b_q = OUh_q \qquad (15)$$

where $h_q = \theta\left(I^U \cdot a_q\right)$ is the output of the hidden layer, and $\theta(.)$ is the sigmoid function. The output weight matrices are calculated using the loss function error of the mean square error, considering that the bottom layer weight matrix U is already known. This is accomplished by using Equation 16 to minimise the average total square error to the learn factor:

$$R = \left| B - U \right|^2 = U_s\left[(B-U)(B-U)^U\right] \qquad (16)$$

As a result, Equation 18 shows if U is constant, the hidden layer values S can be determined, and the upper layer weight matrix P in each module can be approximated using a gradient value calculated in Equation 17:

$$\frac{\sum R}{\sum U} = 2S\left(P^U S - U\right) \qquad (17)$$

As a result, Equation 18 emerges:

$$P = \left(SS^U - U\right) \qquad (18)$$

It should be emphasised that all weight matrices in a deep stacking network module should be empirically configured. This can be done by using random numbers from different distributions to set i or by training a restricted Boltzmann machine (RMB) to set i on its own using contrastive divergence. Gradient descent is used to train the weight matrix i of the DSN in each unit, as indicated in Equation 19.

$$\frac{\sum R}{\sum I} = 2\times\left[s^U e(1-S)^U e\left[S(SU)(US) - U^U(US)\right]\right] \qquad (19)$$

where

$$I^{(p+1)} = I^{(p)} + \gamma \times \frac{\sum R}{\sum I} \qquad (20)$$

where $S = s^U \left(ss^U \right)$, γ is the learning rate, and e indicates element-wise matrix multiplication.

6.5 RESULTS AND DISCUSSION

This section presents an experimental study that was carried out to evaluate the suggested design. Standard gene expression datasets (RNA-Seq) are used in this process. StatFR, RF, and DSN are state-of-the-art algorithms that are compared in our experiments.

6.5.1 Performance Metrics

Unsupervised feature selection methods are suggested as a way to look at data about how genes are expressed. Based on the chosen subset of features, the tasks of predicting cancer in a sample and classifying gene expression data are done. The goal is to find a meaningful feature subset from the original feature subset based on a small number of significant parameters. Feature selection is used for a variety of purposes, including deleting redundant and unnecessary features, reducing dimensionality, enhancing the learning model's performance, and minimising the quantity of data required for learning. The importance of the specified characteristics determines the classification problem's effectiveness. The confusion measure is used to measure the classifier's performance. Based on the specified feature subset, gene expression data are classified. Classification is an unsupervised approach, which means no class information is required [12]. The results of a classification model are used to evaluate its efficiency. In this approach, a variety of cluster validation approaches are used to determine the quality of the classification methods. A few of the performance measures are used to examine the internal and external validation criteria [23]. The performance metrics are calculated based on accuracy, false-positive rate, precision, and recall values. The formulas to calculate the performance metrics are described in the following.

- **Accuracy**—as described in Equation 21, accuracy is the ratio of accurately predicted positive findings to all data. The high accuracy indicates that the classification system is more accurate [24].

$$Accuracy = \frac{TP + TN}{TP + FP + FN + TN} \tag{21}$$

- **False Positive Rate (FPR)**—the amount of false positives is the number of positive values which are expected to be negative. The number of true negative values, which are also anticipated to be negative, is known as the true negative. This metric has a value of 1 to 0. Equation 22 is used to evaluate the false positive rate.

$$FalsePositiveRate\ (FPR) = \frac{FP}{FP + TN} \tag{22}$$

- **Precision**—the precision is described as the proportion of all correct positive predictions to all positive predictions, commonly referred to as positive predictive value (PPV). Specificity has the greatest score of 1 and the worst score of 0. The computation of precision is shown in Equation 23.

$$Precision = \frac{TP}{TP + FP} \tag{23}$$

- **Recall**—the recall is the proportion of accurately estimated positive data to all actual class values. Equation 24 defines the recall value.

$$Recall = \frac{TP}{TP + FN} \tag{24}$$

6.5.2 Analysis and Comparison

The study of RNA-Seq data also examines the ratio of gene expression for several genes at the same time. Due to the limited number of samples and the huge number of genes, analysing gene expression datasets can be difficult. Because the majority of the genes are useless or redundant, feature selection is a crucial guideline for analysing such complicated data. Effective approaches are used to choose features. This study compares the ensemble of three classifier systems with a feature selection algorithm. Our approach is unique in that it is evaluated using an unsupervised deep learning technique. Based on the prior performance of characteristics, a classification method is applied to predict sample outcomes. The experimental methods are evaluated using the confusion matrix, using benchmark datasets such as PRAD, LUAD, BRCA, KIRC, and COAD. Multiple

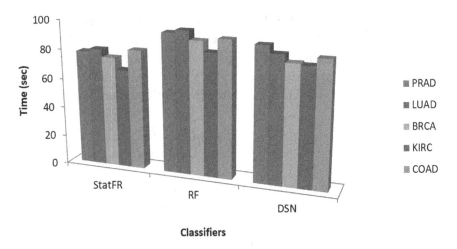

FIGURE 6.3   Comparative analysis of metrics for five RNA sequencing datasets.

classification methods are used to examine the proposed strategy. These experiments are classified based on the evaluation of the selected features; the selection of criteria; and the use of StatFR, RF, and DSN classifiers with a variety of n values. The selected feature subset(s) are the foundation of the first phase of analysis. Figure 6.3 illustrates a performance analysis based on time complexity.

The accuracy of different methods is summarised in the following using RNA-Seq datasets and several classifiers. Table 6.1 demonstrates that the suggested RF architecture outperforms the DSN and StatFR classifiers. Using the recall, FPR, and precision metrics to compare the suggested model to other algorithms, it outperforms them all. In the table, metrics from the confusion matrix are used to compare the proposed method to state-of-the-art algorithms.

Table 6.1 shows the accuracy of the different technique summarised using RNA-Seq datasets and several classifiers. The accuracy of StatFR, RF, and DSN for the PRAD sample is 78%, 94%, and 90%, respectively. On the LUAD sample, the accuracy of StatFR, RF, and DSN is 80%, 96%, and 85%, respectively. On the BRCA sample, StatFR has a 75% accuracy, RF has a 90% accuracy, and DSN has an 80% accuracy. On the KIRC sample, they achieved 67%, 89%, and 79% accuracy. The accuracy of the COAD sample is 81%, 92%, and 84%, respectively. This demonstrates that the suggested RF architecture outperforms the DSN and StatFR classifiers. When evaluating rival algorithms using the recall, FPR, and precision metrics, the

TABLE 6.1   Comparison of Performance Metrics with the Classification Techniques

Classifier Technique	Performance Metric	PRAD (%)	LUAD (%)	BRCA (%)	KIRC (%)	COAD (%)
StatFR	Accuracy	78	80	75	67	81
	FPR	55	63	59	55	64
	Precision	79	69	54	56	60
	Recall	81	79	75	66	71
RF	Accuracy	94	96	90	83	92
	FPR	49	55	53	50	60
	Precision	90	88	79	83	77
	Recall	93	90	81	85	80
DNS	Accuracy	90	85	80	79	84
	FPR	45	50	51	48	57
	Precision	81	75	68	79	71
	Recall	85	83	77	78	80

suggested model outperforms them equally. Table 6.1 compares the proposed approach to state-of-the-art algorithms based on metrics obtained using the confusion matrix. Figure 6.3 illustrates a performance analysis based on time complexity.

6.6 SUMMARY

Gene expression data, such as RNA-Seq datasets, have high dimensionality, which causes a signal-to-noise issue, and they are hard to handle. These high-dimensional data may be processed in one of the following ways: dimensionality reduction using feature extraction techniques like StatFR, RF, and DSN. Depending on the type of original data, either deep learning or machine learning can be used to classify a dataset. High-dimensional datasets are appropriate for machine learning, including RFs; nevertheless, high-dimensional RNA-Seq datasets might not be suitable for a deep learning method since overfitting issues might occur. Machine learning techniques including random forest can be a better alternative for classifying huge RNA-Seq datasets for biomedical research. The RF method may detect features, resulting in more accurate classification and development of significantly important features. The distance between the average of the target and non-target classes, their overlap measure, and the class impurity are statistical characteristics that have an impact on the score values. The result of all categories in each feature is obtained by our method, which is then used to rank the features.

This chapter compares state-of-the-art feature selection techniques by using the top-ranked features to make a heuristic classifier. The experimental findings on certain high-dimensional benchmark data demonstrated that our approach performed better in detecting more important features, resulting in more accurate classifiers with significantly less computing cost. Our study may not be able to manage feature redundancy, since it analyzes each feature independently. Furthermore, it does not examine the impact of other characteristics, making it difficult to determine their relevance or irrelevancy.

REFERENCES

1. Jabeen, A., N. Ahmad, and K. Raza, *Machine learning-based state-of-the-art methods for the classification of RNA-seq data*, in *Classification in BioApps*. 2018, Springer. pp. 133–172.

2. Trapnell, C., et al., *Differential gene and transcript expression analysis of RNA-seq experiments with TopHat and Cufflinks*. Nature Protocols, 2012. **7**(3): pp. 562–578.

3. Zararsiz, G., et al., *Classification of RNA-seq data via bagging support vector machines*. bioRxiv, 2014: p. 007526.

4. Da Silva, R., et al., *BRAF overexpression is associated with BRAF V600E mutation in papillary thyroid carcinomas*. Genetics and Molecular Research, 2015. **14**(2): pp. 5065–5075.

5. Mansoori, E.G., *Using statistical measures for feature ranking*. International Journal of Pattern Recognition and Artificial Intelligence, 2013. **27**(01): p. 1350003.

6. Yoon, H., K. Yang, and C. Shahabi, *Feature subset selection and feature ranking for multivariate time series*. IEEE Transactions on Knowledge and Data Engineering, 2005. **17**(9): pp. 1186–1198.

7. Danaee, P., R. Ghaeini, and D.A. Hendrix. *A deep learning approach for cancer detection and relevant gene identification*. in *Pacific Symposium on Biocomputing 2017*. 2017, World Scientific.

8. Forman, G., *An extensive empirical study of feature selection metrics for text classification*. Journal of Machine Learning Research, 2003. **3**: pp. 1289–1305.

9. Alanni, R., et al., *Deep gene selection method to select genes from microarray datasets for cancer classification*. BMC Bioinformatics, 2019. **20**(1): pp. 1–15.

10. Sabato, S. and S. Shalev-Shwartz, *Ranking categorical features using generalization properties*. Journal of Machine Learning Research, 2008. **9**(6).

11. Schaack, D., M.A. Weigand, and F. Uhle, *Comparison of machine-learning methodologies for accurate diagnosis of sepsis using microarray gene expression data*. PLoS One, 2021. **16**(5): p. e0251800.

12. Al-Obeidat, F., et al., *Gene encoder: A feature selection technique through unsupervised deep learning-based clustering for large gene expression data*. Neural Computing and Applications, 2020: pp. 1–23.

13. Raza, K. and S. Ahmad, *Recent advancement in next-generation sequencing techniques and its computational analysis.* International Journal of Bioinformatics Research and Applications, 2019. **15**(3): pp. 191–220.

14. Ballouz, S., W. Verleyen, and J. Gillis, *Guidance for RNA-seq co-expression network construction and analysis: Safety in numbers.* Bioinformatics, 2015. **31**(13): pp. 2123–2130.

15. Yang, I.S. and S. Kim, *Analysis of whole transcriptome sequencing data: Workflow and software.* Genomics & Informatics, 2015. **13**(4): pp. 119–125.

16. Kashyap, H., et al., *Big data analytics in bioinformatics: A machine learning perspective.* arXiv preprint arXiv:1506.05101, 2015.

17. Yue, T. and H. Wang, *Deep learning for genomics: A concise overview.* arXiv preprint arXiv:1802.00810, 2018.

18. Asuncion, A. and D. Newman, *UCI Machine Learning Repository.* 2007, UCI.

19. Breiman, L., *Bagging predictors.* Machine Learning, 1996. **24**(2): pp. 123–140.

20. Pan, X. and K. Xiong, *PredcircRNA: Computational classification of circular RNA from other long non-coding RNA using hybrid features.* Molecular Biosystems, 2015. **11**(8): pp. 2219–2226.

21. Jiang, P., et al., *MiPred: Classification of real and pseudo microRNA precursors using random forest prediction model with combined features.* Nucleic Acids Research, 2007. **35**(suppl_2): pp. W339-W344.

22. Zhang, J., H. Hadj-Moussa, and K.B. Storey, *Current progress of high-throughput microRNA differential expression analysis and random forest gene selection for model and non-model systems: An R implementation.* Journal of Integrative Bioinformatics, 2016. **13**(5): pp. 35–46.

23. Halim, Z. and J.H. Khattak, *Density-based clustering of big probabilistic graphs.* Evolving Systems, 2019. **10**(3): pp. 333–350.

24. Bhuiyan, M.N.Q., et al., *Transfer learning and supervised classifier based prediction model for breast cancer,* in *Big Data Analytics for Intelligent Healthcare Management.* 2019, Elsevier. pp. 59–86.

CHAPTER 7

Graph Neural Networks for Brain Tumour Segmentation

Nico Loesch and Marc Fischer

7.1 INTRODUCTION

With the advent of machine learning (ML) algorithms capable of detecting patterns in observed data, a new era of automated pattern recognition was initiated. The algorithms are designed to learn from an abundance of examples with differing appearances rather than explicitly programming a machine to solve for a pattern detection task. Traditional ML algorithms were hand-crafted feature selectors designed by domain experts. As a result, the algorithms are intended to solve for a specific task, leading to a reduced potential for generalisation. Convolutional neural networks (CNNs) were introduced to process grid-like data like images, transforming the learning task to an automated end-to-end learning paradigm. Networks are capable of extracting meaningful features without human interaction and domain knowledge. By stacking multiple extraction layers of the CNN, higher-order features can be obtained due to the increased depth of the network. This is usually referred to as deep learning (DL) and constitutes the basis for automated image analysis in many domains (Bishop, 2006; Goodfellow et al., 2016).

Since the discovery of X-rays and subsequently the first medical imaging diagnostic tool by Wilhelm Conrad Röntgen in 1895, more sophisticated imaging methods have been developed and are utilised in clinical routines. Those methods include ultrasound imaging, magnetic resonance imaging

DOI: 10.1201/9781003292357-7

(MRI), computed tomography (CT) and positron emission tomography. These technologies have risen rapidly in importance due to the possibility of detection, characterisation, monitoring, staging and treatment response assessment. However, with the increased number of images to assess highly heterogenous individual diseases, the preservation of an efficient workflow is becoming more and more challenging for radiologists and physicians. As the success of the medical intervention is directly affected by the radiological assessment, precision is essential. However, differences in the assessment between experts can be ascertained due to the diverse manifestation of medical lesions. As a result, automatic analysis tools with a high level of generalisation and reliability are required to assist medical staff in their decision making (Chen & Jain, 2020; Lee & Fujita, 2020; Shen et al., 2017).

Due to the success of DL methods in natural image processing, CNNs are being employed in clinical research in different branches of medicine such as gastroenterology (Le Berre et al., 2020), cardiology (Hannun et al., 2019) and neurology (Zegers et al., 2021). The latter includes the automated analysis of gliomas, a special type of brain tumour. Gliomas are defined by their origin from cells of healthy tissue, such as astrocytomas, oligodendrogliomas or ependymomas. They account for nearly 80% of malignant brain tumours and are classified by the World Health Organization (WHO) based on their malignancy from grade I to grade IV, the glioblastoma. The latter is described by its infiltrative and highly diffusive growth. As patient survival time is directly dependent on the successful safe gross-total resection, accurate boundary margins of the tumour are required. As a result, the traditional image-level classification task, determining what type of lesion is present, must be combined with additional information on localisation (Forst et al., 2014; Pucci et al., 2019; Weller et al., 2015). This is accomplished through the task of semantic segmentation, which groups areas with similar characteristics and thus provides additional information about the lesion in addition to accurate delineation (Goodfellow et al., 2016; Hesamian et al., 2019). Typical DL networks for semantic segmentation are the fully convolutional network by (Long et al., 2015) and its advancement, the U-Net by Ronneberger et al. (2015), with the latter still being used in clinical research due to its remarkable feature extraction capabilities (Feng et al., 2020; Isensee et al., 2021; Zhang et al., 2021).

Many established architectures aiming to solve the segmentation task rely on the aggregation of adjacent pixels in the Euclidean domain by means of the convolution operation and have shown excellent results for different medical datasets (Çiçek et al., 2016; Hesamian et al., 2019; Long et al., 2015; Ronneberger et al., 2015; Zhang et al., 2015). With the emergence of operations targeted to non-Euclidean data in recent years (Bronstein et al., 2016; Kipf & Welling, 2016; Ma et al., 2019; Zhang et al., 2022), the graph structure representing viable information through the interconnection of multiple nodes can be analysed in an automated way. Leveraging regular voxels to the graph domain could be a promising alternative to segmentation methods based on CNNs, as long-range relationships represented by nodes and the connecting edges can be analysed without the loss of localisation. Additionally, graph neural networks (GNNs) are capable of capturing relational information between brain compartments required to learn the global structure of the MRI images (Saueressig et al., 2021).

The contributions of this work are summarised as:

- Development of a novel network architecture comprising a combination of conventional U-Net and Graph U-Net trainable end to end.

- Empirical exploration of a novel architecture to evaluate the advantages of graph operations for medical image segmentation by comparing different graph-specific convolutional operators, pooling methods and normalisation layers.

The subsequent parts of this chapter are organised as follows. Section 7.2 provides an overview of currently employed techniques utilising GNNs for the segmentation of medical images. To get a more in-depth understanding of the GNNs for the task of feature convolution, Section 7.3 introduces the theoretical formulation behind the convolutional operators for unstructured data. The section is followed by a description of the empirical study and its results in Section 7.4. Finally, the chapter closes with a conclusion and an outlook for subsequent studies in the field of brain tumour segmentation in Section 7.5.

7.2 RELATED WORK

The state of the art in medical image segmentation is supervised learning in combination with CNNs in architectures specialised for the task at hand. This nowadays usually includes a modification of the U-Net by

Ronneberger et al. (2015), which is capable of partially retaining locali-sation information through the usage of skip-connections. Modifications extend to the usage of ensembles of this network (Feng et al., 2020; Zhang et al., 2021), multitask learning (Zhao et al., 2020; C. Zhou et al., 2020) and the usage of adversarial training concepts (Myronenko, 2019; Xue et al., 2018), which achieve remarkable results in automatic medical image segmentation.

As soon as the data are no longer grid-like, conventional methods used for CNNs are undefined due the incompatibility of the kernel and the data structure of the input (see Figure 7.1). Methods designed to generalise deep neural networks to the non-Euclidean domain can be summarised by the term *geometric deep learning*. Typical tasks of GNNs focus on node classification, link prediction and clustering. The tasks can be facilitated with a variety of different network structures such as convolutional graph neural networks (ConvGNNs) and graph autoencoders (Bronstein et al., 2016; Liu & Zhou, 2020; Zhang et al., 2022). ConvGNNs redefine the con-volution in terms of spectral and spatial aggregation operators, which are defined in Section 7.3.

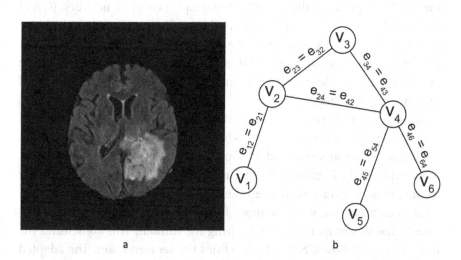

FIGURE 7.1 Comparison of image and graph domain. Individual pixels are arranged in an equidistant spaced grid in images, depicted in (a). Due to the regularity, conventional multi-dimensional convolution can be applied. Graphs contain unstructured nodes V_i connected by respective edges e_{ij} as depicted in (b). This difference to the image domain prevents the usage of the classical convo-lutions as a means of a feature aggregator.

(Garcia-Uceda Juarez et al., 2019) utilise the conventional U-Net structure and replace the bottleneck with a GNN module for the task of airway segmentation from chest CTs. To allow more complex representations, the output features of the CNN encoder are transformed using a two-layered MLP. Instead of following the U-Net structure in the graph branch of the U-Net, the authors stack four layers composed of the GCN (Kipf & Welling, 2016) to extract long-range information beyond the initial neighbourhood. The results evaluated on a private dataset showed that the GNN is capable of segmenting more complete airway trees with fewer trainable parameters whilst upholding similar Dice similarity coefficients (DSCs) for the regions of interest compared to a baseline U-Net.

With respect to automated segmentation of brain tumours relying on GNNs, few approaches are available. Saueressig et al. (2021) build the graph structure required for GNN operations by clustering the brain MRI into a set of k supervoxels based on a trade-off between intensity and spatial information. Each supervoxel represents one node in the graph and is connected with undirected and unweighted edges to r neighbours. This approach is inspired by (Yan et al., 2019), which used a similar technique to segment brain tissue. To obtain features, three GNNs are utilised— the GCN (Kipf & Welling, 2016), the graph attention network (GAT) (Veličković et al., 2018) and GraphSAGE (Hamilton et al., 2017). The latter achieves the best performance on the brain tumour segmentation (BraTS) 2019 dataset and obtains comparable DSCs as the winning model of the previous years' challenge by (Myronenko, 2019) with significantly reduced memory requirements.

Saueressig et al. (2021) subsequently adapted their GNN model and combined it with a conventional CNN to improve upon the coarse predictions due to the supervoxel clustering. The best-performing ConvGNN, the GraphSAGE, is utilised to predict the brain tumour labels, similar to the previous iteration. The reprojection into the voxel-domain is then used in combination with the input features to crop the entire brain volume to the subcompartment containing the tumour. This constitutes the input to the shallow CNN, which refines the segmentation. The adapted approach in combination with a loss function for each network in the model is capable of delineating finer structures in the 2021 iteration of the BraTS challenge.

The aforementioned methods primarily utilise the graph convolutions in a consecutive manner without the usage of pooling operations.

As a result, this study utilises the well-established U-Net structure and combines traditional convolutional layers with graph convolutions in order to evaluate the benefits of the latter. Furthermore, the comparison of different convolutional normalisation layers and pooling operators of the graph domain is performed. Particularly, pooling is required due to the nature of the U-Net and contributes to the novelty of the approach for the task of brain tumour segmentation. Additionally, the superpixel approach by Saueressig et al. (2021) is replaced by conventional convolutional layers, which constitutes an automated end-to-end learning scheme.

7.3 GRAPH NEURAL NETWORKS

This section introduces the theoretical formulation behind the GNN concepts used in this study. It includes a definition of graphs and the historical advancement from spectral to spatial information aggregators in the context of ConvGNNs. The paragraphs predominantly utilise the notation introduced by Wu et al. (2021). For a more in-depth understanding of the network architectures unified as geometric deep learning, information can be found in the respective literature (Bronstein et al., 2016; Liu & Zhou, 2020; Wu et al., 2021; Zhang et al., 2022; J. Zhou et al., 2020).

7.3.1 Definition of Graphs

A graph $G = (\mathcal{V}, \mathcal{E})$ is represented by a set $\mathcal{V}$ composed of $\mathcal{N}$ vertices or nodes and a set of edges $\mathcal{E} \in \mathbb{R}^{N \times N}$. Each edge $e_{uv} = (u, v) \in \mathcal{E}$ is directed from node u to node v. The connectivity of the graph is presented by the adjacency matrix $\mathbf{A} \in \{0,1\}^{N \times N}$ with $\mathbf{A}_{ij} = 1$ if $e_{ij} \in \mathcal{E}$ and $\mathbf{A}_{ij} = 0$ otherwise. If the adjacency matrix is symmetrical, the graph is regarded as *undirected*, as $e_{vu} = e_{vu}$. The degree $d(v)$ of a node depicts the number of neighbours. Both nodes and edges contain features represented by the respective node feature vector $X_v \in \mathbb{R}^C$ is and edge feature vector $X_{vu}^e \in \mathbb{R}^C$ (Liu & Zhou, 2020; Wu et al., 2021; Zhang et al., 2022). To redefine the convolution for the graph domain, spectral and subsequently spatial approaches were developed and are explained in the following sections.

7.3.2 Spectral ConvGNNs

Spectral approaches initially proposed by (Bruna et al., 2014) use the normalised graph Laplacian $\mathbf{L} = \mathbf{I_N} - \mathbf{D}^{-\frac{1}{2}} \mathbf{A} \mathbf{D}^{-\frac{1}{2}}$ to define the convolution operation. $\mathbf{D}_{ii} = \sum\left(\mathbf{A}_{i,j}\right)$ describes the diagonal matrix of node degrees. $\mathbf{L}$ can be refactored as $\mathbf{L} = \mathbf{U}\mathbf{\Lambda}\mathbf{U}^T$ since the normalised Laplacian is symmetric positive semidefinite. This property results from the assumption of an undirected graph leading to a symmetric adjacency matrix. $\mathbf{\Lambda}$ is the spectrum; that is, the diagonal matrix of eigenvalues and $\mathbf{U} = [\mathbf{u}_0, \ldots, \mathbf{u}_{N-1}] \in \mathbb{R}^{N\times N}$ displays the matrix of eigenvectors ordered by eigenvalues. The graph convolution operation $*_G$ of an input signal $\mathbf{X}$ with a learnable filter $\mathbf{g}$ is defined by

$$\mathbf{x} *_G \mathbf{g} = \mathbf{U}\left(\mathbf{U}^T\mathbf{x} \odot \mathbf{U}^T\mathbf{g}\right) \tag{1}$$

with $\odot$ describing the element-wise product. By using a learnable filter $\mathbf{g}_\theta = \mathrm{diag}\left(\mathbf{U}^T\right)$, the convolution defined in Eq. (1) becomes (Liu & Zhou, 2020; Wu et al., 2021; Zhang et al., 2022; J. Zhou et al., 2020):

$$\mathbf{x} *_G \mathbf{g}_\theta = \mathbf{U}\mathbf{g}_\theta\mathbf{U}^T\mathbf{x} \tag{2}$$

As the eigendecomposition of the graph Laplacian is computationally expensive, methods trying to minimise the computational complexity by making several simplifications and approximations were developed (Defferrard et al., 2016; Kipf & Welling, 2016). The reduction of parameters and the introduction of the renormalisation trick of the GCN by Kipf and Welling (2016) reduce the learnable convolution to $\mathbf{x} *_G \mathbf{g}_\theta = \theta\left(\widetilde{\mathbf{D}}^{-\frac{1}{2}} \widetilde{\mathbf{A}}\widetilde{\mathbf{D}}^{-\frac{1}{2}}\right)\mathbf{x}$. However, $\mathbf{g}_\theta$ depends on the composition of the eigenbasis of $\mathbf{L}$, which is based on the adjacency matrix $\mathbf{A}$. As a result, spectral methods impaired in their ability to generalise to graphs with different structures (Liu & Zhou, 2020; Wu et al., 2021; Zhang et al., 2022).

7.3.3 Spatial ConvGNNs

Spatial-based ConvGNNs, on the other hand, define the graph convolution based on a node's spatial relations. Similar to classical CNNs, spatial ConvGNNs aggregate information of a node's neighbourhood $N(v) = \{u \in \mathcal{V} | (i, j) \in \mathcal{E}\}$. By convolving the central node's representation with the features of surrounding nodes, the hidden features of the central node are updated (Liu & Zhou, 2020; Wu et al., 2021).

The framework of message passing neural networks (MPNNs) by Gilmer et al. (2017) unifies several spatial ConvGNNs by defining the graph convolution as a message passing process. To update the hidden node feature vector

$$\mathbf{h}_i^{(k)} = U_k\left(\mathbf{h}_i^{(k-1)}, \sum_{j \in N(i)} M_k\left(\mathbf{h}_j^{(k-1)}, \mathbf{h}_i^{(k-1)}, \mathbf{x}_{ij}^e\right)\right) \quad (3)$$

features of node i are passed along the connecting edges to neighbouring nodes in K steps in order to aggregate information along the way. The message function $M_k(\cdot)$ includes the hidden node feature vector $\mathbf{h}_i^{(k-1)}$ of the node of interest and its adjacent nodes $\mathbf{h}_j^{(k-1)}$ of the previous message passing phase in the message passing phase. Additionally, the edge features $\mathbf{x}_{ij}^e$ are utilised in order to gather information. The final hidden representation is obtained by a vertex update function $U_k(\cdot)$, which is followed either by an output layer or a readout layer for node-level predictions or graph-level predictions, respectively (Gilmer et al., 2017; Wu et al., 2021).

As the traditional MPNN is not capable of aggregating different sets of feature vectors of a node's neighbourhood to different embeddings, Xu et al. (2019) hypothesise that there exists a function $f : X \rightarrow \mathbb{R}$ capable of differentiating between different sets of feature vectors, which can be approximated with a MLP. The graph convolution for a central node of the GIN becomes

$$\mathbf{h}_i^{(k)} = MLP\left(\left(1 + \epsilon^{(k)}\right)\mathbf{h}_i^{(k-1)} + \sum_{j \in N(i)} \mathbf{h}_j^{(k-1)}\right) \quad (4)$$

with $\epsilon^{(k)}$ describing a fixed scalar or learnable parameter (Wu et al., 2021; Xu et al., 2019).

The GAT treats the convolution based on the incorporation of the attention mechanism into the propagation step of the MPNN. It is designed to focus on the most relevant nodes required for predictions and decision making by including learnable weights into the feature aggregation. A network is composed of multiple stacked *graph attention layers*, which compute the attention coefficients α_{ij} of a node pair (i, j) individually as

$$\alpha_{ij}^{(k)} = \frac{\exp\left(\text{LeakyReLU}\left(\mathbf{a}^T\left[\mathbf{Wh}_i^{(k-1)} \| \mathbf{Wh}_j^{(k-1)}\right]\right)\right)}{\sum_{m \in N(i)} \exp\left(\text{LeakyReLU}\left(\mathbf{a}^T\left[\mathbf{Wh}_i^{(k-1)} \| \mathbf{Wh}_m^{(k-1)}\right]\right)\right)}$$

with || describing the operation of concatenation, **W** depicting a weight matrix applied to every node and **a** depicting a learnable weight vector. LeakyReLU represents the leaky rectifier linear unit (ReLU) activation function. The update of the feature vector can be calculated as follows

$$\mathbf{h}_i^{(k)} = \sigma\left(\sum_{j \in N(i)} \propto_{ij}^{(k)} \mathbf{W} \mathbf{h}_j^{(k-1)}\right) 1,$$

with σ depicting the sigmoid activation function. The model is also capable of *multi-head attention*, which performs the N independent attention mechanism, whose hidden features are concatenated to obtain the output feature representation. Furthermore, the computation of the node-neighbour pairs can be computed in parallel, making this operation more efficient (Liu & Zhou, 2020; Veličković et al., 2018; J. Zhou et al., 2020)

7.3.4 Graph U-Net

The network proposed by Gao and Ji (2021) attempts to leverage the traditional U-Net by Ronneberger et al. (2015) to the graph domain. Pooling is performed by a learnable vector projecting all node features onto a one-dimensional feature space, where a top-k pooling operation selects the most import nodes based on their scalar footprint. The scalar projection s_v of the input node feature vector $\mathbf{x}_v$ on a learnable projection vector $\mathbf{p}$ is defined as $s_v = \mathbf{x}_v^T \mathbf{p} / \|\mathbf{x}_v\|$. Upsampling operations take the location of the nodes obtained by the respective top-k pooling operation and replaces the rows of the zero matrix $O_{N \times C}$ by the features of the current layer $\mathbf{H}^{(k)}$, resulting in the feature matrix $\mathbf{X}^{(k+1)}$ of the subsequent layer. For feature aggregation, the GCN by Kipf and Welling (2016) is utilised (Gao & Ji, 2021).

7.3.4.1 Alternative Pooling and Unpooling

As a more static approach towards the learnable pooling and unpooling introduced by Gao and Ji (2021), the pooling method by Simonovsky and Komodakis (2017) and the interpolation method by Qi et al. (2017) are utilised. The former utilises the VoxelGrid algorithm to coarsen the graph structure, which overlays the graph structure with a grid and replaces the nodes by a collective centroid in the form of max-pooling. The interpolation approach by Qi et al. (2017) creates k-nearest neighbours based on the inverse distance weighted average as the distance metric d, such that

$$\mathbf{x}_y = \frac{\sum_{i=1}^{k} w(p_i)\mathbf{x}_i}{\sum_{i=1}^{k} w(p_i)}, \text{ where } w(x_i) = \frac{1}{d(p_y, p_i)^2}$$

with $p_1, \ldots, p_k$ denoting the positions of k-nearest points to the position p_y of node y. $\mathbf{x}_y$ displays the node feature vector of node y, which is interpolated by using the node features of the k-nearest available nodes $\mathbf{X}_i$ (Qi et al., 2017).

7.4 EXPERIMENTS AND RESULTS

7.4.1 Dataset and Experimental Settings

7.4.1.1 Software and Hardware

The proposed framework is based on the machine learning library PyTorch (Paszke et al., 2019), version 1.7.1. The framework considering all graph operations was provided by PyTorch Geometric (Fey & Lenssen, 2019), version 1.6.3. Augmentation and data preprocessing was performed with the TorchIO 0.18.1 package developed by Pérez-García et al. (2021). In order to train the network, a Nvidia GeForce 1080 Ti 11 GB was used.

The dataset used to train the network was obtained by the medical segmentation decathlon (MSD) 2018 (Antonelli et al., 2021) and combines samples of the 2016 and 2017 BraTS challenges (Bakas et al., 2017, 2019; Menze et al., 2015). The 750 samples are composed of clinically acquired pre-operative multimodal MRI scans of glioblastoma and lower-grade glioma. Four different sequences (native T1, contrast-enhanced T1, T2 contrast-enhanced and T2-fluid attenuated inversion recovery) for each individual subject are available. Ground-truth annotations are provided by the organisers of the challenge consisting of necrotic and non-enhancing tumour core (NC), peritumoral oedema and the enhancing tumour (ET), with a fourth label depicting the background (see Figure 7.2). The samples are distributed between a labelled training set consisting of 484 labelled subjects and an unlabelled test dataset. The former was used exclusively in this work due to the requirement of having a ground truth in order to evaluate the performance of the networks, as the challenge has already concluded.

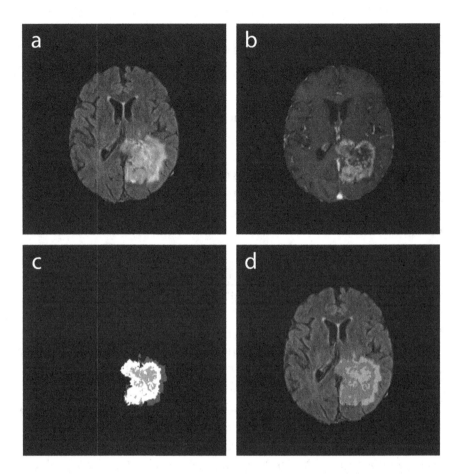

FIGURE 7.2 Visualisation of the MSD dataset. Sample of the MSD dataset depicting one input image with two out of four available MRI sequences ((a) and (b)) for a specific slice. The corresponding label (c) contains four different binary masks for each of the categories of brain tumour present (background, NC, ET and oedema). To visualise the entire label within one image, each binary mask is represented by a different greyscale intensity. Figure (d) depicts the overlay of the label mask onto one of the input images. The labels represent oedema, ET and cystic/NC.

7.4.1.2 Dataset

7.4.1.3 Data Preprocessing

The 484 samples of the original training set were randomly split into separate sets for training (70%), validation (15%) and testing (15%). Preprocessing including augmentation for training samples was composed of a random bias field, z-normalisation, random noise and a random spatial transformation—either affine or elastic deformation. Validation and test subjects were solely normalised with mean and variance of the distribution. The parameters of the transformations were adapted by visual assessment based on the real-life possibility of the proposed augmentations. In order to reduce the computational requirements, patch-based sampling, which randomly extracts patches of size 64×64×64, was utilised for training. For dense inference, a patch-overlap of half the patch size was determined to prevent edge effects.

7.4.1.4 Proposed Model Architecture

The proposed model architecture depicted in Figure 7.3 is a combination of the conventional CNN U-Net by Ronneberger et al. (2015) and the GNN U-Net by Gao and Ji (2021). The number of layers of each U-Net

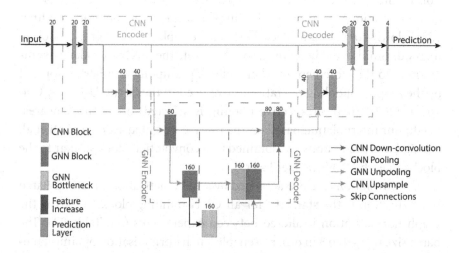

FIGURE 7.3 Proposed network architecture with two stacked U-Nets—one for regular convolution operations (dotted lines at the top-left and top-right) and one for graph convolutions (dotted lines at the bottom-centre) with dCNN = dGNN = 2 (dGNN = 2 is utilised to reserve space for visualisation). Both U-Nets are composed of an encoder and decoder, which share information by skip connections to restore the high-resolution segmentation map. The numerals indicate the number of input feature channels of the respective block. Arrows describe the respective operations, whereas black arrows depict lack of operation and instead the flow of information to the next block. Depicting residual connections of the CNN layers is omitted to preserve a better visibility of the other operations.

can be controlled by the respective hyperparameters dCNN and dGNN. The CNN is utilised to extract meaningful features and to reduce the spatial dimension to enable the memory-intensive graph operations. Each layer of the CNN encoder is composed of two CNN convolutional layers with kernel size of 3 and a residual convolution bypassing the aforementioned blocks (He et al., 2015) and a downsampling operation doubling the feature channels whilst halving the spatial dimensions by utilising a convolutional block with stride 2. The respective CNN decoder performs upsampling by interpolation and utilises the same convolutional blocks with skip-connections from the encoder branch.

In order to generate the graph structure from the image, the k-nearest-neighbour operation provided by PyTorch Geometric was utilised with $k = 4$. The succeeding GNN encoder layers are composed of a pooling operation and a ConvGNN layer. The pooling was either the learnable pooling introduced by Gao and Ji (2021) or a max graph pooling (Simonovsky & Komodakis, 2017). The pooling operation precedes the convolution operation in the GNN U-Net to further reduce the memory footprint of the graph operations—mainly originating from the GAT operator. The final CNN down-convolution block is therefore replaced by a graph pooling method. Similar to the conventional U-Net, the GNN decoder is symmetrical to the aforementioned encoder. Upsampling is either performed by the graph unpooling operation introduced in the Graph U-Net by Gao and Ji (2021) (if the respective pooling is selected) or by the k-nearest neighbour interpolation based on the inverse weighted average of Qi et al. (2017). Final predictions are obtained by a convolution block similar to the blocks in each CNN encoder layer.

All convolutions are pre-activated by a ReLU activation function. Batch normalisation is the standard for all CNN building blocks, whereas the graph normalisation is altered between experiments (see Table 7.1). The batch size was set to 3 in order to enable batch normalisation by simultaneously moderating the required graphics memory.

7.4.1.5 Network Training and Testing

Network training was conducted with six different variations (depicted in Table 7.1) with a baseline as comparison. The baseline replaces the graph operations with a bottleneck layer similar to the implementation by Ronneberger et al. (2015) and is composed of three layers of normal convolutional layers as described in Section 7.1.4. Modifications of the graph network include different ConvGNN layers (GAT, GIN and GCN), the

TABLE 7.1   Test Strategy for the Evaluation of Graph Operations

	Baseline	A	B	C	D	E	F
dCNN	3	2	2	2	2	2	2
dGNN	0	3	3	3	3	3	3
GConv	—	GAT	GAT	GAT	GAT	GIN	GCN
GPool	—	TopK	TopK	Max	Max	Max	Max
GNorm	—	Layer	Batch	Layer	Batch	Batch	Batch

normalisation of the respective layer (batch and layer normalisation) and the pooling method (top-k; Gao & Ji, 2021) with $k = 0.4$ and max-pooling (Simonovsky & Komodakis, 2017). An iterative search was conducted to determine the best-performing GNN with respect to the baseline by comparing conventional performance metrics. This includes overlap-based metrics represented by the DSC and distance-based metrics shown by the 95% Hausdorff distance (HD) (Taha & Hanbury, 2015; Yeghiazaryan & Voiculescu, 2018). Significance is determined by the paired student's t-test (Kalpić et al., 2011) for $p<0.05$ (see Table 7.3). The amount of output feature channels obtained by the feature extraction block preceding the U-Net is set to 20. To find the best parameter vector, the adaptive moment estimation (Adam) optimiser with an initial learning rate of 0.001 in combination with focal loss (Lin et al., 2020) ($\alpha = 0.1$ for background and $\alpha = 0.3$ for each foreground class, $\gamma = 2$) was utilised. The number of maximum epochs was set to 120 and was determined empirically with an early stopping mechanism in place to prevent potential overfitting.

7.4.2 Experimental Results

The baseline CNN U-Net with three layers achieves DSCs of 0.65 ± 0.22 for oedematous tissue, 0.50 ± 0.27 for the NC and 0.70 ± 0.25 for the ET, as depicted in Table 7.2. This represents a good basis for comparison and underlines the capabilities of the basic U-Net architecture, as comparably high scores are achieved without significant modifications. All foreground labels are characterised by high standard deviations (SDs). Similar to the overlap metric, the HD is denoted by rather large SDs. As a result, the 25th, 50th and 75th quartiles were decided upon, as they depict the distribution in greater detail. The respective HD median quartiles for each of the tumour labels are 11.79 mm, 9.90 mm and 3.74 mm. Particularly the 75th percentiles of oedema and NC show significant outliers at 27.39 mm and 32.20 mm, respectively. This shows the heterogeneity of the dataset

TABLE 7.2   DSC of the Test Set Depicted with SD

	Oedema	NC	ET
Baseline	0.65 ± 0.22	0.50 ± 0.27	0.70 ± 0.25
A	0.61 ± 0.23	0.44 ± 0.25	0.68 ± 0.23
B	0.55 ± 0.26	0.41 ± 0.28	0.68 ± 0.26
C	0.54 ± 0.25	0.37 ± 0.24	0.63 ± 0.29
D	0.51 ± 0.27	0.41 ± 0.27	0.59 ± 0.32
E	0.59 ± 0.24	0.46 ± 0.27	0.70 ± 0.24
F	0.48 ± 0.28	0.40 ± 0.28	0.63 ± 0.29

Source: NC: necrotic core, ET: enhancing tumour
All configurations are depicted in Table 7.1.

reported by the organisers (Bakas et al., 2017, 2019), as shown by the results of other contestants (Daza et al., 2021; Isensee et al., 2021), and will be further discussed in Section 7.2.5.

7.4.2.1 How to Normalise the Data?

To investigate the impact of the normalisation method, four experiments with different normalisation strategies are designed. Regarding the learnable pooling iterations (configuration A and B), normalisation presents only a partially significant impact towards accurate boundary delineation. Only the decrease of 6% in mean DSC of the oedema is significant, whereas the other two foreground labels remain within a similar range of means mainly due to the high standard deviation. Additionally, the ET remains stable at 0.68. Regarding the distance-based metric, the outcome appears to be different at first glance, with a decrease in median values for oedema and NC for the iteration with batch normalisation, but significance cannot be obtained. Furthermore, the NC also shows an outlier of the 75th percentile at 66.06 mm.

If one removes the learnable pooling (configuration C and D), a slightly different situation regarding mean and median values of DSCs and HDs can be observed. Whereas layer normalisation achieves significantly higher values in mean DSC for oedema and ET, batch normalisation appears to be superior in the boundary delineation of the NC depicted in Table 7.2 (and significance in Table 7.3). Furthermore, median HDs are reduced significantly for NC and ET for configuration D, which is also reflected in lower

TABLE 7.3   HDs of Test Set Depicted as 25th, 50th and 75th Percentile in Millimetres

	Oedema	NC	ET
Baseline	6.40/11.79/27.39	5.83/9.90/32.20	2.00/3.74/10.63
A	8.06/22.45/53.86	9.06/22.14/42.06	2.45/4.58/15.30
B	7.18/13.45/35.76	6.56/11.18/66.06	2.34/5.00/9.33
C	8.60/15.92/35.85	17.89/65.20/80.65	2.87/7.38/45.13
D	7.28/17.00/51.89	9.06/21.47/67.85	2.24/5.83/13.93
E	7.63/18.11/51.85	6.44/13.34/38.08	2.24/5.44/24.57
F	8.06/20.93/49.32	10.43/31.77/65.12	2.68/6.56/27.24

Source: NC: necrotic core, ET: enhancing tumour
All configurations are depicted in Table 7.1.

25th and 75th percentiles for the same classes. The only class where layer normalisation achieves generally lower distances to the ground-truth is the oedema, which, however, is non-significant despite the reduction of the 75th percentile of 16 mm.

In general, layer normalisation seems to excel in the overlap-based metrics, whereas batch normalisation is generally more accurate in terms of distance to the ground truth. As batch normalisation is reported to require larger batch sizes to calculate the statistics to normalise the input (Ba et al., 2016), the authors recommend the usage of a larger batch size to further utilise the potential this normalisation technique holds. One reason for the obtained results might be that batch normalisation forces a more compact representation resembling the general shape of the lesion. This could lead to misclassification of positive pixels, which reduces the true positive predictions and subsequently impairs the DSC. On the other hand, layer normalisation covers more of the tumour area but results in certain areas with too "narrow" predictions with high distances to the ground-truth mask.

Both normalisation methods are characterised by outliers reflected by large 75th percentiles of the HD and high SD in the DSC. This elevated variance reduces the significance of the obtained results and impedes a clear recommendation for the best normalisation technique. The causes for this are diverse and will be further discussed in Section 7.2.5. To achieve congruence with the normalisation in the CNN layers, the batch normalisation was subsequently utilised as the normalisation of choice, despite the potential drawback of reduced mean DSCs of the general metric of choice to compare segmentation results.

7.4.2.2 The Importance of Pooling

The aforementioned four configurations are also used to determine the most accurate pooling method. The learnable pooling of Gao and Ji (2021) (iteration A and B) and static max-pooling (Simonovsky & Komodakis, 2017) (iteration C and D) are therefore compared to each other.

It is generally observable that the learnable pooling presents a significant benefit over its static counterpart. Regarding the DSC, an average decrease of more than 6% and 4% can be noticed compared to the learnable pooling if the normalisation is kept at layer and batch normalisation, respectively. The sole exception is depicted between configuration B and D regarding the NC with the same mean DSC (0.48) and similar SD at of 0.28 and 0.27, respectively.

The HD follows a similar pattern, with generally reduced distances to the ground truth for learnable pooling. Static pooling achieves on average 75% and 45% higher median HDs for layer and batch normalisation, respectively. However, the only significant deterioration of the static pooling compared to its top-k counterpart can be seen for the NC and the iterations with layer normalisation, as configuration C shows an outlier at 65.20 mm median HD. Despite the absence of significant improvement for the distance-based metric, the reduction in HD interval width due to lower means and fewer outliers cannot be ignored and hints at the superiority of the method.

The observation of better performance through learnable pooling is also reported for conventional CNNs (Li et al., 2019; Zhang & Zhang, 2020). One reason this observation can be made is the additional set of learnable parameters, which are adapted through the gradient of the loss function. The individual pooling layers are therefore adapted in each iteration to select the most important features for the underlying layers. As the projection vector by Gao and Ji (2021) constitutes a simpler approach for learnable pooling, the authors of this chapter expect further improved strategies to arise in the future in order to refine the classification performance of ConvGNNs (Li et al., 2019; Wu et al., 2021; Zhang & Zhang, 2020; J. Zhou et al., 2020).

The reason the projection vector has been replaced by the static max-pooling in configurations D–E is the focus on the graph convolution by forcing a more deterministic behaviour of the pooling layer without additional learnable parameters involved.

7.4.2.3 The Effect of Different Convolutional Operators

To evaluate the performance of different ConvGNNs, the GAT, GIN and GCN were compared (see D–E). The performance of the GIN convolution achieves the highest mean DSC of all graph networks for the ET and the NC. Particularly, the former is equal to the CNN baseline and shows the capabilities of the operation. Furthermore, the GIN operator is significantly better than GAT and GCN for the selected configuration and shows similar mean values to the GAT network with learnable pooling (configuration A), depicted by the non-significant difference in mean DSCs across all classes (see Table 7.3). HDs show again a slightly different picture, with the only significant improvement of the GIN operator being observed for the NC at lower 25th, 50th and 75th percentiles. The incorporation of a learnable mapping function in the case of the GIN increases the representational power of the graph operation, as different features are mapped to different embeddings (Xu et al., 2019).

On the other hand, the spectral GCN attains the lowest mean DSC for oedema and the second-lowest DSC for the remaining classes—NC and ET—at 0.48 ± 0.28, 0.40 ± 0.28 and 0.63 ± 0.29, respectively. Furthermore, the distance-based evaluation illustrates the inferior capability of the method with majorly increased distances of the ground truth to the prediction. The GAT operator is situated between both aforementioned convolutions, with a slightly better accuracy to the GCN mainly regarding the distance-based evaluation, where it occasionally achieves slightly better performance over the GIN, such as in the oedema and the ET, which is, however, non-significant.

This evaluation shows the generally superior performance of spatial-based convolutional operators over their spectral predecessor. The reason behind this accuracy gap is the varying graph structure for different images and manifestations of the disease. This leads to a reduced generalisation capability due to the dependence on the adjacency matrix (Wu et al., 2021; Zhang et al., 2022) and is reported in recent literature (Saueressig et al., 2021). Furthermore, the GAT inherits the potential of global-scale feature aggregation through the attention mechanism, which can be beneficial for context understanding and is utilised in conventional CNN networks (Su et al., 2020; C. Zhou et al., 2020). By utilising multiple attention heads, one might be able to see a performance improvement. Nonetheless, this operator had the highest memory footprint of all tested configurations and not only hindered the usage of multiple attention heads but also the usage of either larger batch sizes or larger patch sizes due maintain the same general configuration for all iterations.

7.4.2.4 Discussion of Graph Operations

In general, the graph operations are slightly inferior to their pure CNN counterpart, the baseline configuration. This is depicted by decreased mean DSCs and increased HDs for the majority of experiments regarding the baseline and is similarly reported in literature (Garcia-Uceda Juarez et al., 2019; Saueressig et al., 2021). One main reason behind this impairment is the limited capability due to the utilisation in combination with a CNN U-Net. This step was required to mitigate the computational requirements of the graph operations initiated by experiments with the GAT. As a result, the graph convolutions only operated on a graph with 32×32×32 nodes for each of the four modalities, which required additional graph pooling to prevent memory excess. The decision to utilise a larger batch size at the expense of a smaller patch size could lead to a reduction in global context required for precise learning. As the preceding U-Net functions similarly to the superpixel strategy of Saueressig et al. (2021), the stacking of several GAT layers to extract more meaningful features might be the cause of the memory excess. This assumption is emphasised by the findings of other publications stating the efficiency of graph operations. Garcia-Uceda Juarez et al. (2019) and Saueressig et al. (2021) limited their approach to using a single graph layer. As deeper graph networks are reported to suffer from a performance drop-off (Li et al., 2018; J. Zhou et al., 2020), a shallower architecture utilising multiple graph layers consecutively will therefore be utilised in subsequent iterations to compare both accuracy and efficiency.

Apart from the aforementioned shortcomings of graph operations, certain configurations achieve remarkable results. Contrast-rich lesions are segmented with similar performance to conventional CNN architectures. The attention mechanism in the GAT is capable of weighting neighbouring nodes based on their importance. By utilising the multi-head capabilities, the weighting is adapted, which could improve the segmentation of smaller-scale lesions such as the NC. The requirement of an injective feature mapping of the GIN operator appears to be beneficial for smaller-scale lesions as features are transformed to distinct embeddings. Finally, the message passing is capable of aggregating information from distant nodes and is efficient in improving scene understanding (Garcia-Uceda Juarez et al., 2019; Saueressig et al., 2021).

7.4.2.5 Insufficient Generalisation Capabilities

In addition to the observations exclusively targeted towards graph operations, high SDs of the DSCs and high 75th percentiles of the HDs are ascertained for all models. This is a definite sign of inferior generalisation performance due to the high variability of the disease. Particularly, the high-grade gliomas encountered in this dataset are characterised by an infiltrative growth with diffuse boundaries. Possible reasons behind this inferior performance are either (a) labelling bias or (b) insufficient model complexity partially caused by limited data samples.

The dataset of the MSD comprises the examples of the 2016 and BraTS challenge (Antonelli et al., 2021). In order to have the best annotations possible, multi-institutional data annotated by various experts following precise guidelines are the cornerstone of the challenge. However, annotation bias due to interobserver experience variations is an empirically observed problem and directly impacts the performance of the supervised segmentation algorithms. Additionally, the authors of the challenge state in the protocol that *radiologic definition of tumour boundaries, especially in such infiltrative tumours as gliomas, is a well-known problem* (Bakas et al., 2017, 2019; Liu et al., 2020; Togao et al., 2016). This underlines the possibility of hypothesis (a), indicated by the omission of samples from the 2016 dataset in the following years of the BraTS challenge with a continuous increase of dataset size since then. One reason behind this change is the obtainment of ground-truth labels by the best-performing segmentation models of previous years (Baid et al., 2021; Bakas et al., 2019), which were refined by medical professionals. Therefore, utilising the recent 2021 iteration of the dataset might provide better ground-truth annotations with, at minimum, coherent labelling.

Furthermore, the comparably small sample size of medical images prevents the development of models with higher capacity, which might be able to detect meaningful features required to successfully delineate highly diffuse lesions. Models with deeper architectures are subject to overfitting and are therefore limited in their predictive capability. The organisers of the most influential brain tumour challenge therefore endeavour to have a larger dataset size with the most significant improvement in quantity in the 2021 iteration to enable more sophisticated DL models (Baid et al., 2021).

The combination of a larger dataset depicting a broader range of inter-subject variance and deeper models is expected to be beneficial for automated detection both in terms of improved accuracy and reduced SDs and has to be shown in subsequent studies with GNNs.

7.5 CONCLUSION AND FUTURE WORK

As brain tumours still present a challenging task for automated segmentation algorithms, more accurate models with improved robustness and generalisation are required to advance towards clinical implementation. As the majority of approaches primarily utilise the well-established CNN, this study explored the potential of graph operations to segment brain tumour images. The shortcomings of the utilised GNNs are the increased memory requirements and slightly reduced performance with respect to smaller-scale subcompartments of brain tumour lesions. Indicated by the emergence of various convolutional operators in the graph domain in recent years (Wu et al., 2021; Zhang et al., 2022), the optimal convolution remains to be determined. This study compared three promising ConvGNNs and showed the potential spatial methods inherit over their spectral counterparts. The predominantly utilised GCN obtains insufficient segmentation results and is outperformed by GIN and GAT. Particularly, the capability of retaining localisation information in deeper layers is beneficial for accurate segmentations (Lu et al., 2019), which is depicted in comparable performance to state-of-the-art models. In particular, the adaptability to diverse graph structures owing to the spatial definition of the convolution has been shown in this study to be significantly beneficial. Both operators inherit unique benefits: The GIN operator is more memory efficient and could be applied to earlier layers in the U-Net architecture. This would provide a higher resolution and more spatial context to the highly expressive operator. On the other hand, the attention mechanism of the GAT operator succeeds in global context learning but is primarily limited by the required convolutional layers to reduce the number of graph nodes due to its higher computational footprint. One solution might be an adapted attention mechanism with an efficient implementation, which will be pursued in subsequent iterations.

In addition, the accuracy of the graph convolution is dependent on the choice of the pooling operator in order to aggregate deeper features with global context. While traditional approaches such as max-pooling are well known and predictable, a focus on learnable downsampling provides another area of research to improve the capabilities of the GNNs (Li et al., 2019; Zhang & Zhang, 2020). This study has shown the potential of a learnable pooling operator, which outperformed the classical max-pooling in the chosen architecture for the GAT. It is expected that other ConvGNNs also benefit from a learnable down-sampling, as is capable of reducing the context to the important features and the adaptation to slight variations of inter-subject manifestations. Subsequent iterations will investigate different pooling operators and their upsampling counterparts to further improve the accuracy and robustness of the graph operations.

Apart from the analysis of the various convolutional and pooling operators, this study also utilised the well-established U-Net architecture for semantic segmentation by combining both conventional and graph sub-networks similar to Saueressig et al. (2021). The initial CNN serves as a feature extractor designed to reduce the computational complexity to facilitate the computationally expensive attention mechanism of the GAT operator whilst simultaneously capturing features from high-resolution layers. It replaces the clustering algorithm proposed by Saueressig et al. (2021) with a learnable feature extractor. As both studies utilise different datasets of the BraTS challenge, an exact comparison can not be facilitated and will be the focus of subsequent studies. However, the proposed architecture shows competitive results with respect to other approaches utilising in the MSD dataset. With the aforementioned improvements indicated by the results of this study, the full potential of graph operations can be analysed to enhance the precision and reliability of highly diffuse brain tumours.

Finally, supervised DL algorithms are reliant on a comprehensive dataset size to achieve the remarkable results reported in the literature (Althnian et al., 2021; Hestness et al., 2017). The organisers of the BraTS challenge aim to continuously improve the dataset regarding quality and quantity by mitigating the labelling bias (Baid et al., 2021). Due to the high labelling cost in medical images, obtaining ground-truth annotations for the substantial variations of medical lesions is a challenging task. Therefore, semi-supervised, transfer or unsupervised learning strategies provide an alternative to classical paradigms by reducing the requirement of ground-truth annotations. Those learning strategies should be investigated in the future in order to overcome the inherent limitations of supervised brain tumour segmentations, bringing DL closer to clinical practice.

REFERENCES

Althnian, A., AlSaeed, D., Al-Baity, H., Samha, A., Dris, A. B., Alzakari, N., Abou Elwafa, A., & Kurdi, H. (2021). Impact of Dataset Size on Classification Performance: An Empirical Evaluation in the Medical Domain. *Applied Sciences, 11*(2), 796. https://doi.org/10.3390/app11020796

Antonelli, M., Reinke, A., Bakas, S., Farahani, K., AnnetteKopp-Schneider, Landman, B. A., Litjens, G., Menze, B., Ronneberger, O., Summers, R. M., van Ginneken, B., Bilello, M., Bilic, P., Christ, P. F., Do, R. K. G., Gollub, M. J., Heckers, S. H., Huisman, H., Jarnagin, W. R., . . . Cardoso, M. J. (2021). The Medical Segmentation Decathlon. *ArXiv:2106.05735 [Cs, Eess]*.

Ba, J. L., Kiros, J. R., & Hinton, G. E. (2016). *Layer Normalization* (Issue arXiv:1607.06450). arXiv. https://doi.org/10.48550/arXiv.1607.06450

Baid, U., Ghodasara, S., Mohan, S., Bilello, M., Calabrese, E., Colak, E., Farahani, K., Kalpathy-Cramer, J., Kitamura, F. C., Pati, S., Prevedello, L. M., Rudie, J. D., Sako, C., Shinohara, R. T., Bergquist, T., Chai, R., Eddy, J., Elliott, J., Reade, W., . . . Bakas, S. (2021). The RSNA-ASNR-MICCAI BraTS 2021 Benchmark on Brain Tumor Segmentation and Radiogenomic Classification. *ArXiv:2107.02314*.

Bakas, S., Akbari, H., Sotiras, A., Bilello, M., Rozycki, M., Kirby, J. S., Freymann, J. B., Farahani, K., & Davatzikos, C. (2017). Advancing the Cancer Genome Atlas Glioma MRI Collections with Expert Segmentation Labels and Radiomic Features. *Scientific Data, 4*(1), 170117. https://doi.org/10.1038/sdata.2017.117

Bakas, S., Reyes, M., Jakab, A., Bauer, S., Rempfler, M., Crimi, A., Shinohara, R. T., Berger, C., Ha, S. M., Rozycki, M., Prastawa, M., Alberts, E., Lipkova, J., Freymann, J., Kirby, J., Bilello, M., Fathallah-Shaykh, H., Wiest, R., Kirschke, J., . . . Menze, B. (2019). *Identifying the Best Machine Learning Algorithms for Brain Tumor Segmentation, Progression Assessment, and Overall Survival Prediction in the BRATS Challenge* (Issue arXiv:1811.02629). arXiv. https://doi.org/10.48550/arXiv.1811.02629

Bishop, C. M. (2006). *Pattern Recognition and Machine Learning*. Springer.

Bronstein, M. M., Bruna, J., LeCun, Y., Szlam, A., & Vandergheynst, P. (2016). *Geometric Deep Learning: Going beyond Euclidean Data*. https://doi.org/10.1109/MSP.2017.2693418

Bruna, J., Zaremba, W., Szlam, A., & LeCun, Y. (2014). *Spectral Networks and Locally Connected Networks on Graphs* (Issue arXiv:1312.6203). arXiv. https://doi.org/10.48550/arXiv.1312.6203

Chen, Y.-W., & Jain, L. C. (Eds.). (2020). *Deep Learning in Healthcare: Paradigms and Applications* (Vol. 171). Springer International Publishing. https://doi.org/10.1007/978-3-030-32606-7

Çiçek, Ö., Abdulkadir, A., Lienkamp, S. S., Brox, T., & Ronneberger, O. (2016). 3D U-Net: Learning Dense Volumetric Segmentation from Sparse Annotation. In S. Ourselin, L. Joskowicz, M. R. Sabuncu, G. Unal, & W. Wells (Eds.), *Medical Image Computing and Computer-Assisted Intervention—MICCAI 2016* (Vol. 9901, pp. 424–432). Springer International Publishing. https://doi.org/10.1007/978-3-319-46723-8_49

Daza, L., Pérez, J. C., & Arbeláez, P. (2021). Towards Robust General Medical Image Segmentation. In M. de Bruijne, P. C. Cattin, S. Cotin, N. Padoy, S. Speidel, Y. Zheng, & C. Essert (Eds.), *Medical Image Computing and Computer Assisted Intervention—MICCAI 2021* (pp. 3–13). Springer International Publishing. https://doi.org/10.1007/978-3-030-87199-4_1

Defferrard, M., Bresson, X., & Vandergheynst, P. (2016). Convolutional Neural Networks on Graphs with Fast Localized Spectral Filtering. *Proceedings of the 30th International Conference on Neural Information Processing Systems,* 3844–3852. IEEE.

Feng, X., Tustison, N. J., Patel, S. H., & Meyer, C. H. (2020). Brain Tumor Segmentation Using an Ensemble of 3D U-Nets and Overall Survival Prediction Using Radiomic Features. *Frontiers in Computational Neuroscience, 14,* 25. https://doi.org/10.3389/fncom.2020.00025

Fey, M., & Lenssen, J. E. (2019). *Fast Graph Representation Learning with PyTorch Geometric* (Issue arXiv:1903.02428). arXiv. https://doi.org/10.48550/arXiv.1903.02428

Forst, D. A., Nahed, B. V., Loeffler, J. S., & Batchelor, T. T. (2014). Low-Grade Gliomas. *The Oncologist, 19*(4), 403–413. https://doi.org/10.1634/theoncologist.2013-0345

Gao, H., & Ji, S. (2021). Graph U-Nets. *IEEE Transactions on Pattern Analysis and Machine Intelligence,* 1–1. https://doi.org/10.1109/TPAMI.2021.3081010

Garcia-Uceda Juarez, A., Selvan, R., Saghir, Z., & de Bruijne, M. (2019). A Joint 3D UNet-Graph Neural Network-Based Method for Airway Segmentation from Chest CTs. In H.-I. Suk, M. Liu, P. Yan, & C. Lian (Eds.), *Machine Learning in Medical Imaging* (pp. 583–591). Springer International Publishing. https://doi.org/10.1007/978-3-030-32692-0_67

Gilmer, J., Schoenholz, S. S., Riley, P. F., Vinyals, O., & Dahl, G. E. (2017). Neural Message Passing for Quantum Chemistry. *Proceedings of the 34th International Conference on Machine Learning—Volume 70,* 1263–1272. IEEE.

Goodfellow, I., Bengio, Y., & Courville, A. (2016). *Deep Learning.* The MIT Press.

Hamilton, W., Ying, Z., & Leskovec, J. (2017). Inductive Representation Learning on Large Graphs. In I. Guyon, U. V. Luxburg, S. Bengio, H. Wallach, R. Fergus, S. Vishwanathan, & R. Garnett (Eds.), *Advances in Neural Information Processing Systems* (Vol. 30). Curran Associates, Inc.

Hannun, A. Y., Rajpurkar, P., Haghpanahi, M., Tison, G. H., Bourn, C., Turakhia, M. P., & Ng, A. Y. (2019). Cardiologist-Level Arrhythmia Detection and Classification in Ambulatory Electrocardiograms Using a Deep Neural Network. *Nature Medicine, 25*(1), 65–69. https://doi.org/10.1038/s41591-018-0268-3

He, K., Zhang, X., Ren, S., & Sun, J. (2015). *Deep Residual Learning for Image Recognition* (Issue arXiv:1512.03385). arXiv. https://doi.org/10.48550/arXiv.1512.03385

Hesamian, M. H., Jia, W., He, X., & Kennedy, P. (2019). Deep Learning Techniques for Medical Image Segmentation: Achievements and Challenges. *Journal of Digital Imaging, 32*(4), 582–596. https://doi.org/10.1007/s10278-019-00227-x

Hestness, J., Narang, S., Ardalani, N., Diamos, G., Jun, H., Kianinejad, H., Patwary, M. M. A., Yang, Y., & Zhou, Y. (2017). *Deep Learning Scaling Is Predictable, Empirically* (Issue arXiv:1712.00409). arXiv. https://doi. org/10.48550/arXiv.1712.00409

Isensee, F., Jaeger, P. F., Kohl, S. A. A., Petersen, J., & Maier-Hein, K. H. (2021). nnU-Net: A Self-Configuring Method for Deep Learning-Based Biomedical Image Segmentation. *Nature Methods, 18*(2), 203–211. https://doi.org/ 10.1038/s41592-020-01008-z

Kalpić, D., Hlupić, N., & Lovrić, M. (2011). Student's t-Tests. In M. Lovric (Ed.), *International Encyclopedia of Statistical Science* (pp. 1559–1563). Springer. https://doi.org/10.1007/978-3-642-04898-2_641

Kipf, T. N., & Welling, M. (2016). *Semi-Supervised Classification with Graph Convolutional Networks*. https://doi.org/10.48550/arXiv.1609.02907

Le Berre, C., Sandborn, W. J., Aridhi, S., Devignes, M.-D., Fournier, L., Smaïl-Tabbone, M., Danese, S., & Peyrin-Biroulet, L. (2020). Application of Artificial Intelligence to Gastroenterology and Hepatology. *Gastroenterology, 158*(1), 76–94.e2. https://doi.org/10.1053/j.gastro.2019.08.058

Lee, G., & Fujita, H. (Eds.). (2020). *Deep Learning in Medical Image Analysis: Challenges and Applications* (Vol. 1213). Springer International Publishing. https://doi.org/10.1007/978-3-030-33128-3

Li, Q., Han, Z., & Wu, X.-M. (2018). *Deeper Insights into Graph Convolutional Networks for Semi-Supervised Learning* (Issue arXiv:1801.07606). arXiv. https://doi.org/10.48550/arXiv.1801.07606

Li, S., Li, W., Cook, C., Zhu, C., & Gao, Y. (2019). A Fully Trainable Network with RNN-based Pooling. *Neurocomputing, 338,* 72–82. https://doi.org/10.1016/j. neucom.2019.02.004

Lin, T.-Y., Goyal, P., Girshick, R., He, K., & Dollar, P. (2020). Focal Loss for Dense Object Detection. *IEEE Transactions on Pattern Analysis and Machine Intelligence, 42*(2), 318–327. https://doi.org/10.1109/TPAMI.2018.2858826

Liu, Z., Tong, L., Jiang, Z., Chen, L., Zhou, F., Zhang, Q., Zhang, X., Jin, Y., & Zhou, H. (2020). *Deep Learning Based Brain Tumor Segmentation: A Survey*. https://doi.org/10.48550/ARXIV.2007.09479

Liu, Z., & Zhou, J. (2020). Introduction to Graph Neural Networks. *Synthesis Lectures on Artificial Intelligence and Machine Learning, 14*(2), 1–127. https://doi.org/10.2200/S00980ED1V01Y202001AIM045

Long, J., Shelhamer, E., & Darrell, T. (2015). Fully Convolutional Networks for Semantic Segmentation. *ArXiv:1411.4038 [Cs]*.

Lu, Y., Chen, Y., Zhao, D., & Chen, J. (2019). Graph-FCN for Image Semantic Segmentation. In H. Lu, H. Tang, & Z. Wang (Eds.), *Advances in Neural Networks—ISNN 2019* (pp. 97–105). Springer International Publishing. https://doi.org/10.1007/978-3-030-22796-8_11

Ma, F., Gao, F., Sun, J., Zhou, H., & Hussain, A. (2019). Attention Graph Convolution Network for Image Segmentation in Big SAR Imagery Data. *Remote Sensing, 11*(21), 2586. https://doi.org/10.3390/rs11212586

Menze, B. H., Jakab, A., Bauer, S., Kalpathy-Cramer, J., Farahani, K., Kirby, J., Burren, Y., Porz, N., Slotboom, J., Wiest, R., Lanczi, L., Gerstner, E., Weber, M.-A., Arbel, T., Avants, B. B., Ayache, N., Buendia, P., Collins, D. L., Cordier, N., . . . Van Leemput, K. (2015). The Multimodal Brain Tumor Image Segmentation Benchmark (BRATS). *IEEE Transactions on Medical Imaging*, 34(10), 1993–2024. https://doi.org/10.1109/TMI.2014.2377694

Myronenko, A. (2019). 3D MRI Brain Tumor Segmentation Using Autoencoder Regularization. In A. Crimi, S. Bakas, H. Kuijf, F. Keyvan, M. Reyes, & T. van Walsum (Eds.), *Brainlesion: Glioma, Multiple Sclerosis, Stroke and Traumatic Brain Injuries* (Vol. 11384, pp. 311–320). Springer International Publishing. https://doi.org/10.1007/978-3-030-11726-9_28

Paszke, A., Gross, S., Massa, F., Lerer, A., Bradbury, J., Chanan, G., Killeen, T., Lin, Z., Gimelshein, N., Antiga, L., Desmaison, A., Köpf, A., Yang, E., DeVito, Z., Raison, M., Tejani, A., Chilamkurthy, S., Steiner, B., Fang, L., . . . Chintala, S. (2019). PyTorch: An Imperative Style, High-Performance Deep Learning Library. In *Proceedings of the 33rd International Conference on Neural Information Processing Systems*. Curran Associates Inc.

Pérez-García, F., Sparks, R., & Ourselin, S. (2021). TorchIO: A Python Library for Efficient Loading, Preprocessing, Augmentation and Patch-Based Sampling of Medical Images in Deep Learning. *Computer Methods and Programs in Biomedicine*, 208, 106236. https://doi.org/10.1016/j.cmpb.2021.106236

Pucci, C., Martinelli, C., & Ciofani, G. (2019). Innovative Approaches for Cancer Treatment: Current Perspectives and New Challenges. *Ecancermedicalscience*, 13, 961. https://doi.org/10.3332/ecancer.2019.961

Qi, C. R., Yi, L., Su, H., & Guibas, L. J. (2017). PointNet++: Deep Hierarchical Feature Learning on Point Sets in a Metric Space. *Proceedings of the 31st International Conference on Neural Information Processing Systems*, 5105–5114.

Ronneberger, O., Fischer, P., & Brox, T. (2015). U-Net: Convolutional Networks for Biomedical Image Segmentation. *ArXiv:1505.04597 [Cs]*.

Saueressig, C., Berkley, A., Kang, E., Munbodh, R., & Singh, R. (2021). Exploring Graph-Based Neural Networks for Automatic Brain Tumor Segmentation. In J. Bowles, G. Broccia, & M. Nanni (Eds.), *From Data to Models and Back* (pp. 18–37). Springer International Publishing. https://doi.org/10.1007/978-3-030-70650-0_2

Saueressig, C., Berkley, A., Munbodh, R., & Singh, R. (2021). *A Joint Graph and Image Convolution Network for Automatic Brain Tumor Segmentation*. https://doi.org/10.48550/arXiv.2109.05580

Shen, D., Wu, G., & Suk, H.-I. (2017). Deep Learning in Medical Image Analysis. *Annual Review of Biomedical Engineering*, 19(1), 221–248. https://doi.org/10.1146/annurev-bioeng-071516-044442

Simonovsky, M., & Komodakis, N. (2017). *Dynamic Edge-Conditioned Filters in Convolutional Neural Networks on Graphs* (Issue arXiv:1704.02901). arXiv. https://doi.org/10.48550/arXiv.1704.02901

Su, R., Liu, J., Zhang, D., Cheng, C., & Ye, M. (2020). Multimodal Glioma Image Segmentation Using Dual Encoder Structure and Channel Spatial Attention Block. *Frontiers in Neuroscience, 14.*

Taha, A. A., & Hanbury, A. (2015). Metrics for Evaluating 3D Medical Image Segmentation: Analysis, Selection, and Tool. *BMC Medical Imaging, 15*(1), 29. https://doi.org/10.1186/s12880-015-0068-x

Togao, O., Hiwatashi, A., Yamashita, K., Kikuchi, K., Mizoguchi, M., Yoshimoto, K., Suzuki, S. O., Iwaki, T., Obara, M., Van Cauteren, M., & Honda, H. (2016). Differentiation of High-Grade and Low-Grade Diffuse Gliomas by Intravoxel Incoherent Motion MR Imaging. *Neuro-Oncology, 18*(1), 132–141. https://doi.org/10.1093/neuonc/nov147

Veličković, P., Cucurull, G., Casanova, A., Romero, A., Liò, P., & Bengio, Y. (2018). *Graph Attention Networks* (Issue arXiv:1710.10903). arXiv. https://doi.org/10.48550/arXiv.1710.10903

Weller, M., Wick, W., Aldape, K., Brada, M., Berger, M., Pfister, S. M., Nishikawa, R., Rosenthal, M., Wen, P. Y., Stupp, R., & Reifenberger, G. (2015). Glioma. *Nature Reviews Disease Primers, 1*(1), 15017. https://doi.org/10.1038/nrdp.2015.17

Wu, X., Bi, L., Fulham, M., Feng, D. D., Zhou, L., & Kim, J. (2021). Unsupervised Brain Tumor Segmentation Using a Symmetric-Driven Adversarial Network. *Neurocomputing, 455,* 242–254. https://doi.org/10.1016/j.neucom.2021.05.073

Wu, Z., Pan, S., Chen, F., Long, G., Zhang, C., & Yu, P. S. (2021). A Comprehensive Survey on Graph Neural Networks. *IEEE Transactions on Neural Networks and Learning Systems, 32*(1), 4–24. https://doi.org/10.1109/TNNLS.2020.2978386

Xu, K., Hu, W., Leskovec, J., & Jegelka, S. (2019). *How Powerful Are Graph Neural Networks?* (Issue arXiv:1810.00826). arXiv. https://doi.org/10.48550/arXiv.1810.00826

Xue, Y., Xu, T., Zhang, H., Long, L. R., & Huang, X. (2018). SegAN: Adversarial Network with Multi-scale L1 Loss for Medical Image Segmentation. *Neuroinformatics, 16*(3–4), 383–392. https://doi.org/10.1007/s12021-018-9377-x

Yan, Z., Youyong, K., Jiasong, W., Coatrieux, G., & Huazhong, S. (2019). Brain Tissue Segmentation Based on Graph Convolutional Networks. *2019 IEEE International Conference on Image Processing (ICIP),* 1470–1474. https://doi.org/10.1109/ICIP.2019.8803033

Yeghiazaryan, V., & Voiculescu, I. (2018). Family of Boundary Overlap Metrics for the Evaluation of Medical Image Segmentation. *Journal of Medical Imaging, 5*(01), 1. https://doi.org/10.1117/1.JMI.5.1.015006

Zegers, C. M. L., Posch, J., Traverso, A., Eekers, D., Postma, A. A., Backes, W., Dekker, A., & van Elmpt, W. (2021). Current Applications of Deep-Learning in Neuro-Oncological MRI. *Physica Medica, 83,* 161–173. https://doi.org/10.1016/j.ejmp.2021.03.003

Zhang, W., Li, R., Deng, H., Wang, L., Lin, W., Ji, S., & Shen, D. (2015). Deep Convolutional Neural Networks for Multi-Modality Isointense Infant Brain Image Segmentation. *NeuroImage, 108,* 214–224. https://doi.org/10.1016/j.neuroimage.2014.12.061

Zhang, X., & Zhang, X. (2020). Global Learnable Pooling With Enhancing Distinctive Feature for Image Classification. *IEEE Access*, 8, 98539–98547. https://doi.org/10.1109/ACCESS.2020.2997078

Zhang, Y., Zhong, P., Jie, D., Wu, J., Zeng, S., Chu, J., Liu, Y., Wu, E. X., & Tang, X. (2021). Brain Tumor Segmentation From Multi-Modal MR Images via Ensembling UNets. *Frontiers in Radiology*, 1, 704888. https://doi.org/10.3389/fradi.2021.704888

Zhang, Z., Cui, P., & Zhu, W. (2022). Deep Learning on Graphs: A Survey. *IEEE Transactions on Knowledge and Data Engineering*, 34(1), 249–270. https://doi.org/10.1109/TKDE.2020.2981333

Zhao, Y.-X., Zhang, Y.-M., & Liu, C.-L. (2020). Bag of Tricks for 3D MRI Brain Tumor Segmentation. In A. Crimi & S. Bakas (Eds.), *Brainlesion: Glioma, Multiple Sclerosis, Stroke and Traumatic Brain Injuries* (pp. 210–220). Springer International Publishing. https://doi.org/10.1007/978-3-030-46640-4_20

Zhou, C., Ding, C., Wang, X., Lu, Z., & Tao, D. (2020). One-Pass Multi-Task Networks With Cross-Task Guided Attention for Brain Tumor Segmentation. *IEEE Transactions on Image Processing*, 29, 4516–4529. https://doi.org/10.1109/TIP.2020.2973510

Zhou, J., Cui, G., Hu, S., Zhang, Z., Yang, C., Liu, Z., Wang, L., Li, C., & Sun, M. (2020). Graph Neural Networks: A Review of Methods and Applications. *AI Open*, 1, 57–81. https://doi.org/10.1016/j.aiopen.2021.01.001

CHAPTER 8

Biomedical Data Analytics and Visualisation—A Methodological Framework

Quang Vinh Nguyen, Zhonglin Qu,
Chng Wei Lau, Yezihalem Tegegne, Jesse Tran,
Girija Rani Karetla, Paul J. Kennedy,
Simeon J. Simoff, and Daniel R. Catchpoole

8.1 INTRODUCTION

Biomedical information covers a wide range of data that relate to human health. Biomedical data are usually large and complex in terms of volume and multivariate, multiscale, and highly connected and dependent relationships among the data items. Such data might hold important clues regarding diseases, offer knowledgeable insights, or present how individual patients respond differently to treatment strategies. Extracting and interactively presenting the knowledge in a meaningful and understandable way would embrace the complexity of the data for personalised medicine.

To handle such large amounts of often complex information, computational analysis, such as machine learning, including deep learning and statistical methods, has often been used to generate knowledge or conclusions. As biomedical data usually have a large number of dimensions,

 DOI: 10.1201/9781003292357-8

computational analysis methods often require feature selection methods (such as those in the review in [1]) or dimensionality reduction methods (such as in [2–4]). These methods reduce the complexity of multi-dimensionality, reveal patterns, and identify relevant subpopulations in the data. Unfortunately, the lack of ground truth and expert validation or verification would dampen the effectiveness and usefulness of the computational analysis processes [5]. It is essential to integrate visualisation and human involvement to accelerate discovery and trust in the analyses [6] and computational analysis model(s) [7].

Visualisation has been recognised and extensively used in biomedical research and applications, such as in 3D genomics, single-cell RNA sequencing, and extended reality, including augmented reality-assisted surgery, protein structures, and many more, such as those in the survey works [6, 8]. However, visualisation is often underutilised by clinicians and domain experts. A bad or complex visualisation might generate errors or high cognitive overhead that could lead to faulty cognitive processing of the data. Alternatively, an oversimple visualisation may miss important relationships within the data and insightful information. Therefore, it is crucial to reduce such errors by improving the meaningfulness of data visualisation, visual perception and trust with training, and end-user involvement in the development.

Visualising data, especially in the health area, is not an easy task. It involves careful design principles such that it not only focuses on the aesthetics or wow factor but can also show and review the patterns or (ab)normalities in complex and high-dimensional biomedical data. Thus, an effective visualisation would need to use familiar or intuitive visual conventions so that the presented information can be perceived better with less cognitive overload and higher acceptability by the end users. In addition, better training given to the end-user could improve the understanding, perception, interpretability, and acceptability of the visualisation.

Interaction and exploration are crucial components that are usually integrated within visualisations [6]. Interaction is helpful in exploration and deep analysis during the analysis stage. The mantra "overview first, zoom and filter, details on demands" [9] is often adopted, for example, the novel visual analytic platform that integrates domain knowledge and comprehensive capability to enable seamless interaction and exploration of genomic data from the processed patient population space to individual genes of interest [10–12]. Users can also interact and manipulate raw data on demand for better verification and trust while simplifying the visualisation with focused knowledge on the processed data.

Biomedical data visualisation can also go beyond ordinary displays by utilising a wide range of other platforms, such as portable devices [13] and immersive platforms, such as large and high-resolution displays [14], and extended reality, including virtual reality (VR) and augmented reality (AR), as discussed in the recent survey paper [15]. The adaptation of emerging technologies into data analytics and visualisation could pave new ways to see and interact with information from a different angle not possible in a typical display. Unfortunately, at the current stage, most visualisation works in immersive environments focus on volume rendering and modelling computed tomography (CT) (such as [16]), magnetic resonance imaging (MRI) data (such as [17]), pain treatment (such as [18]), rehabilitation (such as summarised in [19]), and other applications (such as those discussed in [20]). It is noticeable in recent work pioneering in VR technologies with well-known visualisation, interaction, design principles, and computational analysis models that create a comprehensive platform for analysing biomedical and genomic data [21].

This chapter provides an introductory tutorial on how biomedical data can be analysed and visualised. We present a diagram to illustrate the necessary steps in the process, emphasising the required components in the analytics cycle. The chapter shows computational analytics methods for biomedical data, including regression, clustering, deep learning, and dimensionality reduction. We discuss interactive visualisation techniques that can be used in biomedical data analytics.

8.2 FRAMEWORK OF BIOMEDICAL DATA ANALYTICS

As biomedical data are large and complex, a single process or method alone can effectively handle and extract knowledge from big data. Effective analytics require multiple components, as shown in Figure 8.1, where the data for knowledge can be gained through pre-observation, computational analytics, and visual analytics.

8.2.1 Pre-Observation

Pre-observation is an important first step for collecting, cleaning, and performing preliminary data analysis to ensure the quality and consistency of the data. The data collection process is usually required when the data are retrieved from heterogeneous sources with different formats

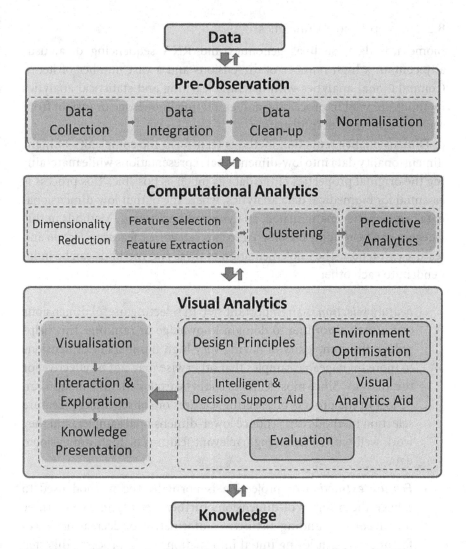

FIGURE 8.1 The analytics flow for biomedical data, adapted from [11, 21].

and sometimes very large to achieve all at once. Thus, it is vital to have a mechanism to collect the required information and transfer it into readable form for further processing. Preliminary data processing and analysis, including data integration, data clean-up, and normalisation, can be applied to produce the centralised datasets with minimal variations, errors, or noises.

8.2.2 Computational Analytics

Biomedical data, such as genomics and RNA sequencing data, usually contain a high number of dimensions and a vast number of items. Computational analytics with machine learning and statistical analytics methods are vital in processing and extracting knowledge or insight from such vast amounts of information.

Dimensionality reduction methods transform the complexity of high-dimensionality data into low-dimensional representations while maintaining the original properties of the data as much as possible. This process is essential for biomedical data analytics, where the output low-dimensional data can be better manipulated, analysed, and presented. Methods in this category can be roughly classified into two categories: feature *selection* and feature *extraction*. The implementation of these two methods can be independent to each other.

- *Feature selection* is an important step in selecting useful dimensions or features according to domain knowledge or ranking. This helps reduce the complexity of having very high numbers of dimensions to more manageable samples that otherwise may not be effective for the analysis. Since most features could be excluded, information can be lost in the process of selecting features or subset choices. Feature selection methods can produce lower-dimensional samples, and they work well within removing irrelevant features or high-dimensional data.

- *Feature extraction* or projection is normally the method used to reduce the number of dimensions further, usually to two or three dimensions, by finding distinctive, informative, or decreasing sets of features without losing initial information in the process. This step is usually useful when the number of dimensions is very large, such as tens of thousands in genomics data in which, unfortunately, the number of chosen features in the feature selection process is usually still high for effective visualisation or decision-making. Feature extraction methods are also useful in revealing relevant subpopulations in the data.

Clustering is a process that automatically partitions the data into logical groups before analysing them. Thus, clustering methods are very useful for exploring the projected data where the clusters or logical groups can be identified and presented to the end users. Clustering methods can be used independently or together with manual selection in the data analysis.

Predictive analytics use additional machine learning methods and models to support the computational analytics process. This step provides further predictive capabilities and relevant features in the processed data. For example, we could use predictive analytics to derive a treatment suggestion for a new patient based on an existing large cohort.

8.2.3 Visual Analytics

After the computational analytics process, the processed data are usually in the form of low-dimensional data (usually in 2D or 3D), with the possibility of having relational structures (such as trees, graphs, or networks) and clusters. Visual analytics and visualisation are essential tools to allow the users to view and interact with the processed data as well as the original data in an interpretable way. This component usually includes visualisation, interaction and exploration, and knowledge representation. Visual analytics allow domain users to analyse the data further using humans' powerful visual perception, pattern recognition, and analytical strength, where the knowledge discovery process can be easily amendable to biomedical experts with their domain knowledge. It is also helpful to build trust and validate the outputs from the computational analytics methods.

The visualisation provides methods to show the processed data in 2D, 3D, or higher-dimensional spaces, where supporting filtering, interaction, and manipulation activities is also integrated into the visualisation. Domain analysts interact and explore the complex information in a simplified and intuitive way to make further discoveries in the data and gain better insight into the data and their structures. With the discovery of new knowledge, the analyst can evaluate, refine, go beyond, and ultimately confirm hypotheses built from previous iterations. The discovery and knowledge gained from this can also be presented in simplified forms for final and executive decisions.

Supporting theory and methods for effective visual analytics are useful in the process, including design principles, environment optimisation, intelligent and decision support aid, visual analytics aid, and evaluation. Design principles are essential to the presentation and user interface to ensure simplicity, well-structured presentation, and visibility of the visualisation. Environment optimisation is critical to large-scale or emerging environments where the users could not view or interact with the information in an ordinary way, such as in VR and AR [21]. Intelligent and decision support and visual analytics aids that use artificial intelligence, such as game theory, can also be used to support and improve the analytics. Validation and evaluation should also co-operate throughout the development process together with the domain experts to improve the acceptability and perceived utility of the visual analytics. We next discuss the popular and useful analytics methods for biomedical data.

8.3 COMPUTATIONAL ANALYTICS METHODS

8.3.1 Feature Selection

Feature selection is one of the most useful keys to the computational analytics of biomedical data. It allows the selection of useful features from the very high-dimensional data with tens of thousands of dimensions (see Figure 8.2 for the flow diagram). Significant research efforts have contributed rich, innovative methods and algorithms in the field, such as in recent reviews [1, 22, 23]. Popular feature selection methods are classified into three main categories (filters, wrappers, and embedded), along with extended categories (including hybrid, ensemble, and integrative) [22].

- Filter methods are early feature selection processes that can work independently with a subsequent learning algorithm. The features are selected based on one or more defined evaluation criteria or a score to assess the degree of relevance of each characteristic [24]. This approach has been adopted in practice thanks to its simplicity and low computational cost.

- Wrapper methods use a classifier to evaluate the relevance of a subset of characteristics, such as accuracy, within a trained predictive model, such as using a deep learning model [11] based on the random forest classifier [25]. Although this approach is superior to the filter

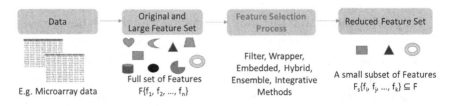

FIGURE 8.2 The feature selection flow diagram.

methods in terms of better accuracy performance, wrapper methods are much more computationally expensive due to the high computational cost of the predictive models.

- Embedded methods utilise the speedy quality of filter methods and the high accuracy of wrapper methods by reducing the degree of overfitting or variance of a model by adding more bias. In this approach, the learning is not separated from the feature selection process, such as using the Monte Carlo feature selection algorithm and an optimised SVM classifier method to identify the significant features [26]. Also, to improve speed, an embedded method might use an advanced computational strategy, such as distributed implementation using the MapReduce K-nearest neighbour classifier for microarray leukaemia data [27].

- Hybrid methods combine multiple feature selection methods (filters, wrappers, and embedded) in the same process to achieve better outcomes, which makes hybrid methods popular in the biomedical data analytics community. Particularly, hybrid methods have been used to build support vector machine (SVM)–based classifiers for better outcomes, such as by combining the Monte-Carlo feature selection method with the incremental feature selection method to effectively identify important features for five different cancers [28] or by iteratively adjusting a bound on the l1-norm of the classifier vector [29].

- Ensemble methods improve the approximation of the subset of features by combining independent feature subsets. For example, Farid et al. combine traditional k-means and similarity-based clustering methods for ensemble clustering of complex genomic data [30], and Hogan *et al.* use a mix of real and synthetic data to improve the effectiveness of parallel ensembles of simpler classifiers (particularly random forests) for Next Generation Sequencing data.

- Integrative methods work by integrating external data or additional selection method(s) during the feature selection process. For example, Zhu et al. applied a low-rank constraint on the weight coefficient matrix before decomposing it into two low-rank matrices to identify the relationships between genetic features and brain image features [31]. This method achieved higher accuracy in finding important single-nucleotide polymorphisms (SNPs) in the Alzheimer's Disease

Neuroimaging Initiative dataset. Other methods can work on multiple data sources using pre-processing followed by the fireflies gravitational ant colony optimisation (FGACO) process to select optimised features for further predictive analytics [32].

8.3.2 Feature Extraction

Feature extraction or projection methods can be applied to project the data to a low number of dimensions, usually in two-dimensional or three-dimensional spaces, such as in [12, 21, 33]. This process is very useful for capturing the complexity of high-dimensional data as well as unveiling patterns or relevant subpopulations in the data, such as in flow cytometry data [2, 34] and single-cell RNA sequencing data [35, 36]. Dimensionality reduction methods can be classified as linear or non-linear approaches, such as the popular methods in the comprehensive review of Maaten *et al.* [37].

- Linear projection methods, including principal component analysis (PCA), are a classic and effective approach to support high-throughput cell biology [38, 39]. They can be effectively used in the early stage of the process to provide proper preliminary analysis before using advanced dimensionality reduction methods [33, 40]. Nevertheless, the linear project approach does not usually capture well the non-linear relationships which are usually presented in the biomedical data [2, 35],

- Non-linear projection methods, such as in [33, 41], are more popular in advanced biomedical data analysis, where they can usually reveal more meaningful subpopulations in the data [2]. Among them, t-SNE [3] (or viSNE [35]) and UMAP [4, 36] are the common techniques for the biomedical data [2, 33, 40]. These methods can capture well the distinctive cell populations in the cytometry and transcriptomic data, which is crucial for analysis and decision-making, such as the abnormal T-cell populations in routine clinical flow cytometry data [42]. UMAP methods outperform t-SNE methods in run time while producing similar and compacted sub-populations in the outcomes [33, 36, 40]. In addition, the computational time of the UMAP process could be improved to 100 times faster using the GPU optimisation [34].

8.3.3 Clustering

Clustering methods as an unsupervised learning approach have been popularly used in biomedical research, such as for the analysis of gene expression, genomic data, MRI images, and more. Clustering methods for biomedical data can be roughly classified into different types, such as hierarchical clustering, centroid-based clustering, fuzzy clustering, neural network-based clustering, kernel learning-based clustering, and density-based clustering, as comprehensively reviewed in [43]. Among them, some methods could perform better than others in one or more applications; however, no particular method has outperformed all others across all criteria or datasets [44].

Hierarchical clustering methods group similar objects into hierarchies of clusters using a nested partitioning approach in either agglomerative (bottom-up) or divisive (top-down) approaches. Hierarchical clustering has been used widely in microarray gene expression data, such as [45, 46].

K-means clustering is a classic and well-known partition-based algorithm, one of the most popular methods in the biomedical field. This method is easy to implement, is fast and efficient, and can partition data into K clusters. This method has mostly been used in gene expression data, such as [47], and medical image processing, such as [48, 49]. Other methods can also overcome the local minima search problem in K-means-based algorithms with global or approximately global optimisation, such as the ant colony optimisation algorithm [50].

Fuzzy clustering, also called soft clustering or soft k-means, allows data points to belong to multiple clusters rather than just one. Methods in this approach can be used to establish the relationships between genes and multiple functional categories or the conditional coregulation of gene expression data, such as in recent work [51].

Neural network–based clustering methods adopt the concept of competitive learning to identify clusters in the data, which is reviewed in [52]. Recent procedures also apply deep neural network(s) to integrate the learning process to improve the cluster results, such as in the review in [53]. This approach has been used popularly in magnetic resonance imaging, such as in [54] and gene expression data analysis [55].

Density-based clustering works by detecting areas where points are concentrated and the emptiness or sparse of the surrounding space. DBSCAN [56, 57] is a popular method in this direction that has a high ability to discover arbitrarily shaped clusters and is robust towards outlier detection or noise. It has been used in gene clustering, such as [58]; biomedical images, such as [59]; and other applications.

8.4 VISUAL ANALYTICS AND VISUALISATION

Scatterplots, charts, histograms, boxplots, heat-maps, parallel coordinates, Venn diagrams, and network visualisation are common methods used to identify patterns or trends, such as in recent reviews [6, 8]. Visual analytics tools often combine multiple visualisation methods to present the same data from the overview and details. By providing multiple views of the same data in different ways, we can gain better insights and utilise the strengths of different visualisations (see Figure 8.3).

8.4.1 Scatter Plot or Dot Plot Visualisation

Scatter plots or dot plots use dot points or small shapes to represent values of pair-wise variables on the X-axis and Y-axis. This method is useful in the early stage of the analysis, which can reveal the correlations and patterns of data items in 2D or 3D space and provide a snapshot of the large information. Visual properties, such as colours, shapes, sizes, and glyphs,

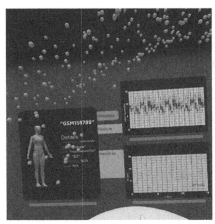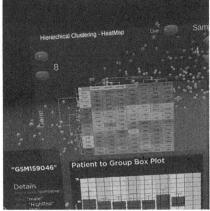

FIGURE 8.3 In this example, multiple visualisation methods are used to support the exploration and analysis of biomedical data in VR space with a VROOM system [21], including scatter plots with regression, box plots, bar charts, and heat maps with hierarchical clustering.

can also be used to provide additional information on higher dimensional data [60]. Multiple scatter plots, such as linkable scatter plots [61] and scatter plot matrices, are also used in biomedical data visualisation, such as flow cytometry data analytics [62]. By integrating a comprehensive interaction and flexibility in showing concurrently the projected outputs and selected markers and side scatters, linkable scatter plots enable effective analysis and discovery of chronic lymphocytic leukaemia diagnoses from the flow cytometry data [34].

Figure 8.4 presents two examples of scatterplot visualisation of biomedical data. Figure 8.4a shows a single scatter plot of the patient cohorts whose additional attributes are mapped with the visual mapping. Figure 8.4b shows the linkable and concurrent scatterplot views of the processed and raw data. Specifically, the top-left panel presents the UMAP projection [4] outcome in 2D space, and other panels present selected markers and side scatters of the original flow cytometry data. Brushing and linking are also used to highlight the chosen items (red dots) across all panels, where the user can learn and validate the outcome of the processed data from the raw data. The red dots are the cancer cells which are identified from the computational analytics.

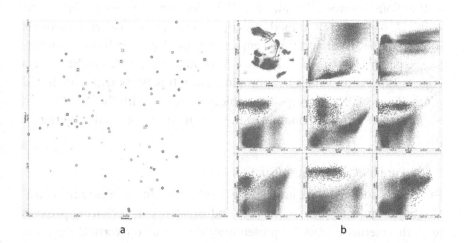

a   b

FIGURE 8.4 An example of scatterplots of biomedical data, in which a) a single scatterplot view on a small set of the patient populations in the genetic similarity space after the analysis and b) multiple scatterplots with brushing and linking are used to show both processed and selected original flow cytometry data for better comparison and validation.

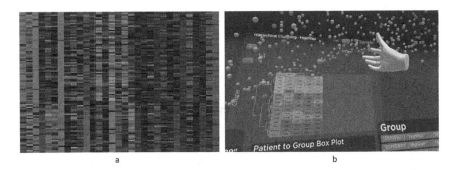

FIGURE 8.5   An example of heat-map visualisations of biomedical data: a) a heat-map view of 30 selected genes (columns) across the 100 patients where we can see expression values are varied across the population and b) a hierarchical clustered heat-map visualisation on a small sample of patients and genes in 3D virtual space, VROOM [21].

8.4.2 Heat-Map Visualisation

Heat-map visualisation uses colours to encode data values in tabular tiles, which is excellent in showing variance and correlations across several variables as well as revealing patterns. Heat-map methods are widely used in the bioinformatics domain, especially for gene expression data (such as in [14, 63]). Heat-map methods can also integrate clustering methods (such as in [6, 21]) or additional enrichment (such as in [64]) to reveal better the patterns in the data. Figure 8.5a shows an example of a heat-maps of gene expression values of approximately 100 patients with 20 selected genes. Figure 8.5b integrates hierarchical clustering with the heat-maps to illustrate better the distribution of the heat-maps in the small selection of patients and genes.

8.4.3 Parallel Coordinate Visualisation

Parallel coordinates have gradually gained popularity in biomedical visu-alisation thanks to their robustness and capability in reviewing patterns [65]. The methods work by presenting data points on vertical axes and then connecting the points by straight lines or curves (see Figure 8.6). Enhancements such as edge bundling, transparency, sampling, and inter-actions are commonly employed to overcome overcrowding in the data with high dimensions or large volumes [66].

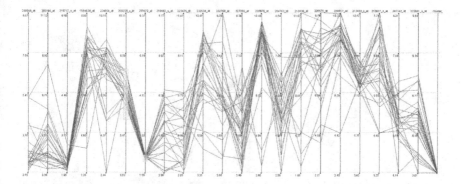

FIGURE 8.6   An example of parallel coordinates on genomic data. The visualisation presents the gene expression values for 20 selected genes for the patient cohort. A filter is also used to reduce the complexity of the visualisation by limiting the ranges of gene expression values on two genes.

8.4.4 Network or Graph Visualisation

Networks, graphs, and pathways are also used in biomedical applications, where they are used to assist predictive analytics and exploratory analysis, such as in [6]. Network visualisation in biomedical applications normally uses a spring-embedded or force-directed method [67, 68] and other forces to lay out the relational structures. Although these methods are relatively computationally expensive, they are widely used in practice due to their ability to show the connectivity of information, as well as the robustness in generating good layouts and easy implementation. Edge bundling is also applied to visualisations to enhance the visibility of the flows in the networks. Figure 8.7 shows an example of a network of genetic similarities between individual patients in the cohort (left), where the gene expression values can be further explored in the heat-map visualisation (right) [14].

8.4.5 Tailored Visualisation

With the rapid growth of biomedical data in terms of volume and complexity, tailored visualisation and advanced interactive visualisation methods and technologies have been developed to meet the need for data exploration, allowing targeted questions to be addressed. A tailored visualisation includes suitable designs usually in cooperation with multiple visual expressiveness and interaction methods to work best on specific types of datasets in cooperation with domain users and the application

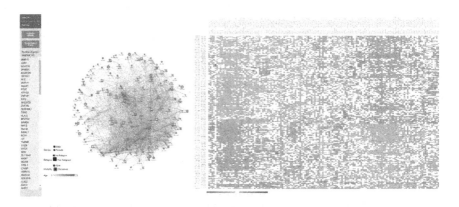

FIGURE 8.7   An example of a network visualisation of patients, visually display-ing their genetic similarity (genetic similar patients are located closer together), and the heat-map view (right panel) further explains the genetic values of the patients for better comparison [14].

context [6]. Tailored visualisation for biomedical data is covered by the work of Nguyen et al. addressing the genomics data analytics for acute lymphoblastic leukaemia and rhabdomyosarcoma data [10–12]. The authors integrated various visualisation methods, including 3D scatter plots, to provide an overview of the entire population in the similarity space of their genetic information, together with the ability to drill down interactively to the genes of interest via heat-maps and dot-plot views for better comparison of the selected patients. The later work VROOM [21] expanded this further in the extended reality environment that included further refinement and extension of the visual design, visual analytics capability, and interaction.

8.4.6 Emerging Technologies

Emerging technologies, such as extended reality, including VR and AR, have been gradually adopted in biomedical visualisation, such as those in recent reviews [15, 69]. Such technologies have been used in disease diag-nostics, volume rendering and modelling of computed tomography and magnetic resonance imaging data [16, 70], patient care, and pain treatment [19, 71]. Beyond personal computer platforms, genomics data analytics has been adopted in different platforms, including mobile devices [72, 73] and large immersive environments [14, 74] where game technology is used to support fluid and seamless analytics in the 3D environment.

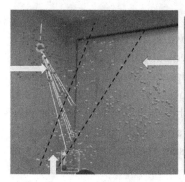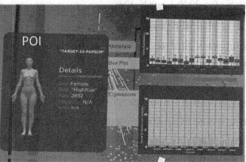

FIGURE 8.8   An example of VROOM in AR environment where i) the left figure shows the overview of the entire patient cohort in the genetic similarity space, and ii) show the visual analytics panels at a navigational stage of a selected patient.

Recently, VR and AR have been adopted in biomedical data visualisation, such as CellexalVR [75], StarMap [76], MinOmics [77], BioVR [78], and VROOM [21]. CellaxalVR presents single-cell RNA sequencing data by coupling multiple statistical data analytics methods in the tool, while StarMap focuses on a mobile web browser on a VR-enabled smartphone. On the other hand, MiniOmics and BioVR utilise UnityMol to manipulate and visualise biomedical data; particularly, MiniOmics focuses on proteomic and transcriptomic data, and BioVR focuses on DNA and RNA sequences, multi-omics data, and protein structures.

Noticeably, virtual reality for the observation of oncology models is new work that employs multiple state-of-the-art methods to provide a complete and comprehensive tool for analysing cancer patient cohorts in both VR and AR environments, including computational analytics, 3D visualisation, audio and design principals, and visual analytics [21]. The tool cleverly employs classical charts in its visual presentation (such as scatter plots, descriptive statistical information, linear regression, box plots, and heat-maps) to provide familiar and meaningful views to the domain users. Game theory is also used to provide intelligent assistance in the decision-making process. Figure 8.3 shows an example of VROOM at an explorational stage in a VR environment (Oculus Quest), and Figure 8.8 shows an example of VROOM in an AR environment (Microsoft HoloLens) on acute myeloid leukaemia (AML) data.

8.5 CONCLUSION

This chapter proposes a structured framework for the application with methods and techniques to support biomedical data analytics. We provide a complete analytical cycle and a comprehensive review of supporting methods that are required in these processes. This chapter works as a guideline for researchers and students who want to study and develop methods in both computational analytics and visual analytics to tackle the complexity of biomedical data and present the outcomes in easy and meaningful ways.

REFERENCES

1. B. Remeseiro and V. Bolon-Canedo, "A review of feature selection methods in medical applications," *Computers in Biology and Medicine*, vol. 112, p. 103375, 2019. https://doi.org/10.1016/j.compbiomed.2019.103375.
2. A. Konstorum, N. Jekel, E. Vidal, and R. Laubenbacher, "Comparative analysis of linear and nonlinear dimension reduction techniques on mass cytometry data," *bioRxiv*, p. 273862, 2018. https://doi.org/10.1101/273862.
3. L. V. D. Maaten and G. Hinton, "Visualizing data using t-SNE," *Journal of Machine Learning Research*, vol. 9, pp. 2579–2605, 2008.
4. L. McInnes, J. Healy, and J. Melville, "UMAP: Uniform manifold approximation and projection for dimension reduction," *arXiv:1802.03426 [stat.ML]*, 2018.
5. D. Cirillo and A. Valencia, "Big data analytics for personalized medicine," *Current Opinion in Biotechnology*, vol. 58, pp. 161–167, 2019. https://doi.org/10.1016/j.copbio.2019.03.004.
6. S. I. O'Donoghue, B. F. Baldi, S. J. Clark, A. E. Darling, J. M. Hogan, S. Kaur, L. Maier-Hein, D. J. McCarthy, W. J. Moore, E. Stenau, J. R. Swedlow, J. Vuong, and J. B. Procter, "Visualization of biomedical data," *Annual Review of Biomedical Data Science*, vol. 1, pp. 275–304, 2018. https://doi.org/10.1146/annurev-biodatasci-080917-013424.
7. Z. Qu, Y. Zhou, Q. V. Nguyen, and D. R. Catchpoole, "Using visualization to illustrate machine learning models for genomic data," in *Proceedings of the Australasian Computer Science Week Multiconference*, ACM Press, 2019, pp. 1–8.
8. G. A. Pavlopoulos, D. Malliarakis, N. Papanikolaou, T. Theodosiou, A. J. Enright, and I. Iliopoulos, "Visualizing genome and systems biology: Technologies, tools, implementation techniques and trends, past, present and future," *GigaScience*, vol. 4, pp. 1–27, 2015.
9. B. Shneiderman, "The eyes have it: A task by data type taxonomy for information visualizations," in *IEEE Symposium on Visual Languages*, Washington, 1996, pp. 336–343.
10. Q. V. Nguyen, A. Gleeson, N. Ho, M. L. Huang, S. Simoff, and D. Catchpoole, "Visual analytics of clinical and genetic datasets of acute lymphoblastic leukaemia," in *2011 International Conference on Neural Information Processing (ICONIP 2011)*, Shanghai, 2011, pp. 113–120.

11. Q. V. Nguyen, N. H. Khalifa, P. Alzamora, A. Gleeson, D. Catchpoole, P. J. Kennedy, and S. Simoff, "Visual analytics of complex genomics data to guide effective treatment decisions," *Journal of Imaging*, vol. 2, pp. 1–17, 2016. https://doi.org/10.3390/jimaging2040029.

12. Q. V. Nguyen, G. Nelmes, M. L. Huang, S. Simoff, and D. Catchpoole, "Interactive visualization for patient-to-patient comparison," *Genomics & Informatics*, vol. 12, pp. 263–276, 2014.

13. Q. V. Nguyen, C. W. Lau, Z. Qu, M. L. Huang, S. Simoff, and D. R. Catchpoole, "A mobile tool for interactive visualisation of genomics data," in *9th International Conference on Information Technology in Medicine and Education (ITME)*, Hangzhou, 2018, pp. 688–697. https://doi.org/10.1109/itme.2018.00158.

14. A. Brunker, D. Catchpoole, P. Kennedy, S. Simoff, and Q. V. Nguyen, "Two-dimensional immersive cohort analysis supporting personalised medical treatment," in *2019 23rd International Conference in Information Visualization-Part II*, Adelaide, 2019, pp. 34–41. https://doi.org/10.1109/iv-2.2019.00016.

15. Z. Qu, C. W. Lau, S. J. Simoff, P. J. Kennedy, Q. V. Nguyen, and D. R. Catchpoole, "Review of innovative immersive technologies for healthcare applications," *Innovations in Digital Health, Diagnostics, and Biomarkers*, vol. 2, pp. 27–39, 2022.

16. C. Calì, J. Baghabra, D. J. Boges, G. R. Holst, A. Kreshuk, F. A. Hamprecht, M. Srinivasan, H. Lehväslaiho, and P. J. Magistretti, "Three-dimensional immersive virtual reality for studying cellular compartments in 3D models from EM preparations of neural tissues," *The Journal of Comparative Neurology*, vol. 524, pp. 23–38, 2016. https://doi.org/10.1002/cne.23852

17. D. B. Douglas, C. A. Wilke, J. D. Gibson, J. M. Boone, and M. Wintermark, "Augmented reality: Advances in diagnostic imaging," *Multimodal Technologies and Interaction*, vol. 1, p. 29, 2017.

18. J. Llobera, M. González-Franco, D. Perez-Marcos, J. Valls-Solé, M. Slater, and M. V. Sanchez-Vives, "Virtual reality for assessment of patients suffering chronic pain: A case study," *Experimental Brain Research*, vol. 225, pp. 105–117, 2013. https://doi.org/10.1007/s00221-012-3352-9.

19. K. E. Laver, B. Lange, S. George, J. E. Deutsch, G. Saposnik, and M. Crotty, "Virtual reality for stroke rehabilitation," *Cochrane Database of Systematic Reviews*, vol. 11, 2016. https://doi.org/10.1002/14651858.CD008349.pub4

20. Z. Qu, C. W. Lau, D. R. Catchpoole, S. Simoff, and Q. V. Nguyen, "Intelligent and immersive visual analytics of health data," in *Advanced Computational Intelligence in Healthcare*, Maglogiannis, I., Brahnam, S., and Jain, L. C., Eds., ed Cham: Springer, 2020, pp. 29–44. https://doi.org/10.1007/978-3-662-61114-2_3.

21. C. W. Lau, Z. Qu, D. Draper, R. Quan, A. Braytee, A. Bluff, D. Zhang, A. Johnston, P. J. Kennedy, S. Simoff, Q. V. Nguyen, and D. Catchpoole, "Virtual reality for the observation of oncology models (VROOM): immersive analytics for oncology patient cohorts," *Scientific Reports*, vol. 12, p. 11337. https://doi.org/10.1038/s41598-022-15548-1.

22. K. Tadist, S. Najah, N. S. Nikolov, F. Mrabti, and A. Zahi, "Feature selection methods and genomic big data: A systematic review," *Journal of Big Data* vol. 6, 2019. https://doi.org/10.1186/s40537–019–0241–0.

23. L. Wang, Y. Wang, and Q. Chang, "Feature selection methods for big data bioinformatics: A survey from the search perspective," *Methods*, vol. 111, pp. 21–31, 2016. https://doi.org/10.1016/j.ymeth.2016.08.014.

24. S. Landset, T. M. Khoshgoftaar, A. N. Richter, and T. Hasanin, "A survey of open source tools for machine learning with big data in the Hadoop ecosystem," *Journal of Big Data*, vol. 2, 2015. https://doi.org/10.1186/s40537–015–0032–1.

25. L. Breiman, "Random forests," *Machine Learning*, vol. 45, pp. 5–32, 2001.

26. Y. H. Zhang, Y. Hu, Y. Zhang, L. D. Hu, and X. Kong, "Distinguishing three subtypes of hematopoietic cells based on gene expression profiles using a support vector machine," *Biochimica et Biophysica Acta (BBA)—Molecular Basis of Disease*, vol. 1864, pp. 2255–2265, 2018. https://doi.org/10.1016/j.bbadis.2017.12.003.

27. M. Kumar, N. K. Rath, and S. K. Rath, "Analysis of microarray leukemia data using an efficient MapReduce-based K-nearest neighbor classifier," *Journal of Biomedical Informatics*, vol. 60, pp. 395–409, 2016. https://doi.org/10.1016/j.jbi.2016.03.002.

28. S. Wang and Y. Cai, "Identification of the functional alteration signatures across different cancer types with support vector machine and feature analysis," *Biochimica et Biophysica Acta: Molecular Basis of Disease*, vol. 1864(6 Pt B), pp. 2218–2227, 2018. https://doi.org/10.1016/j.bbadis.2017.12.026.

29. B. Ghaddar and J. Naoum-Sawaya, "High dimensional data classification and feature selection using support vector machines," *European Journal of Operational Research*, pp. 993–1004, 2018.

30. D. M. Farid, A. Nowe, and B. Manderick, "A feature grouping method for ensemble clustering of high-dimensional genomic big data," in *2016 Future Technologies Conference (FTC)*, San Francisco, CA, 2016, pp. 260–268.

31. X. Zhu, H. Suk, H. Huang, and D. Shen, "Low-rank graph-regularized structured sparse regression for identifying genetic biomarkers," *IEEE Transactions on Big Data*, vol. 3, pp. 405–414, 2017.

32. O. AlFarraj, A. AlZubi, and A. Tolba, "Optimized feature selection algorithm based on fireflies with gravitational ant colony algorithm for big data predictive analytics," *Neural Computing and Applications*, vol. 31, 2019.

33. M. D. Luecken and F. J. Theis, "Current best practices in single-cell RNA-seq analysis: A tutorial," *Molecular Systems Biology*, vol. 15, p. e8746, 2019.

34. Y. Tegegne, Z. Qu, Y. Qian, and Q. V. Nguyen, "Parallel nonlinear dimensionality reduction using GPU acceleration," in *Australasian Conference on Data Mining*, Springer, 2021, pp. 3–15.

35. E.-A. D. Amir, K. L. Davis, M. D. Tadmor, E. F. Simonds, J. H. Levine, S. C. Bendall, D. K. Shenfeld, S. Krishnaswamy, G. P. Nolan, and D. Pe'er, "VISNE enables visualization of high dimensional single-cell data and reveals phenotypic heterogeneity of leukemia," *Nature Biotechnology*, vol. 31, pp. 545–552, 2013. https://doi.org/10.1038/nbt.2594.

36. E. Becht, L. McInnes, J. Healy, C.-A. Dutertre, I. W. H. Kwok, L. G. Ng, F. Ginhoux, and E. W. Newell, "Dimensionality reduction for visualizing single-cell data using UMAP," *Nature Biotechnology*, vol. 37, pp. 38–44, 2018. https://doi.org/10.1038/nbt.4314.

37. L. Van Der Maaten, E. Postma, and J. V. D. Herik, "Dimensionality reduction: A comparative," *Journal of Machine Learning Research*, vol. 10, p. 13, 2009.

38. L. Haghverdi, F. Buettner, and F. J. Theis, "Diffusion maps for high-dimensional single-cell analysis of differentiation data," *Bioinformatics*, vol. 31, pp. 2989–2998, 2015.

39. M. Ringnér, "What is principal component analysis?," *Nature Biotechnology*, vol. 26, pp. 303–304, 2008.

40. M. D. Luecken and F. J. Theis, "Current best practices in single-cell RNA-seq analysis: A tutorial," *Molecular Systems Biology*, vol. 15, p. e8746, 2019. https://doi.org/10.15252/msb.20188746.

41. J. A. Lee and M. Verleysen, *Nonlinear Dimensionality Reduction*, vol. 1. Springer, 2007.

42. J. A. DiGiuseppe, J. L. Cardinali, W. N. Rezuke, and D. Pe'er, "PhenoGraph and viSNE facilitate the identification of abnormal T-cell populations in routine clinical flow cytometric data," *Cytometry B—Clinical Cytometry*, vol. 94, pp. 588–601, 2018.

43. R. Xu and D. C. Wunsch, "Clustering algorithms in biomedical research: A review," *IEEE Reviews in Biomedical Engineering*, vol. 3, pp. 120–154, 2010.

44. C. Wiwie, J. Baumbach, and R. Röttger, "Comparing the performance of biomedical clustering methods," *Nature Methods*, vol. 12, pp. 1033–1038, 2015.

45. A. Alizadeh, M. Eisen, R. Davis, C. Ma, I. S. Lossos, A. Rosenwald, J. C, D. Botstein, P. O. Brown, and L. M. Staudt, "Distinct types of diffuse large B-cell lymphoma identified by gene expression profiling," *Nature*, vol. 403, pp. 503–511, 2000.

46. J. Herrero, A. Valencia, and J. N. Dopazo, "A hierarchical unsupervised growing neural network for clustering gene expression patterns," *Bioinformatics*, vol. 17, pp. 126–136, 2001. https://doi.org/10.1093/bioinformatics/17.2.126.

47. S. Tavazoie, J. D. Hughes, M. J. Campbell, R. J. Cho, and G. M. Church, "Systematic determination of genetic network architecture," *Nature Genetics*, vol. 22, pp. 281–285, 1999.

48. H. Ng, S. Ong, K. Foong, P.-S. Goh, and W. Nowinski, "Medical image segmentation using k-means clustering and improved watershed algorithm," in *2006 IEEE Southwest Symposium on Image Analysis and Interpretation*, 2006, pp. 61–65.

49. N. Dhanachandra, K. Manglem, and Y. J. Chanu, "Image segmentation using K-means clustering algorithm and subtractive clustering algorithm," *Procedia Computer Science*, vol. 54, pp. 764–771, 2015.

50. M. Dorigo, M. Birattari, and T. Stutzle, "Ant colony optimization," *IEEE Computational Intelligence Magazine*, vol. 1, pp. 28–39, 2006.

51. P. S. Raja, "Brain tumor classification using a hybrid deep autoencoder with Bayesian fuzzy clustering-based segmentation approach," *Biocybernetics and Biomedical Engineering*, vol. 40, pp. 440–453, 2020.

52. K.-L. Du, "Clustering: A neural network approach," *Neural Networks*, vol. 23, pp. 89–107, 2010.

53. M. R. Karim, O. Beyan, A. Zappa, I. G. Costa, D. Rebholz-Schuhmann, M. Cochez, and S. Decker, "Deep learning-based clustering approaches for bioinformatics," *Briefings in Bioinformatics*, vol. 22, pp. 393–415, 2020. https://doi.org/10.1093/bib/bbz170.

54. B. Ragupathy and M. Karunakaran, "A deep learning model integrating convolution neural network and multiple kernel K means clustering for segmenting brain tumor in magnetic resonance images," *International Journal of Imaging Systems and Technology*, vol. 31, pp. 118–127, 2021.

55. O. Ahmed and A. Brifcani, "Gene expression classification based on deep learning," in *2019 4th Scientific International Conference Najaf (SICN)*, 2019, pp. 145–149.

56. M. Ester, H.-P. Kriegel, J. Sander, and X. Xu, "A density-based algorithm for discovering clusters in large spatial databases with noise," in *Proceedings of the Second International Conference on Knowledge Discovery and Data Mining (KDD-96)*, AAAI Press, 1996, pp. 226–231.

57. E. Schubert, J. Sander, M. Ester, H. P. Kriegel, and X. Xu, "DBSCAN revisited, revisited: Why and how you should (Still) use DBSCAN," *ACM Transaction on Database Systems*, vol. 42, p. Article 19, 2017.

58. D. R. Edla, P. K. Jana, and I. S. Member, "A prototype-based modified DBSCAN for gene clustering," *Procedia Technology*, vol. 6, pp. 485–492, 2012.

59. M. E. Celebi, Y. A. Aslandogan, and P. R. Bergstresser, "Mining biomedical images with density-based clustering," in *International Conference on Information Technology: Coding and Computing (ITCC'05)-volume II*, 2005, pp. 163–168.

60. Q. V. Nguyen, M. L. Huang, and S. Simoff, "Using hybrid scatterplots for visualizing multi-dimensional data," in *Integrating Artificial Intelligence and Visualization for Visual Knowledge Discovery*, Kovalerchuk, B., Nazemi, K., Andonie, R., Datia, N., and Banissi, E., Eds., ed Cham: Springer International Publishing, 2022, pp. 517–538. https://doi.org/10.1007/978–3–030-93119-3_20.

61. Q. P. V. Nguyen, S. Simoff, Y. Qian, and M. L. Huang, "Deep exploration of multidimensional data with linkable scatterplots," in *9th International Symposium on Visual Information Communication and Interaction*, Dallas, TX: ACM Press, 2016, pp. 43–50. https://doi.org/10.1145/2968220.2968248.

62. S. C. Bendall, R. M. Nolan, and G. P. Chattopadhyay, "A deep profiler's guide to cytometry," *Trends Immunology*, vol. 33, pp. 323–332, 2012.

63. Q. V. Nguyen, P. Alzamora, N. Ho, M. L. Huang, S. Simoff, and D. Catchpoole, "Unlocking the complexity of genomic data of RMS patients through visual analytics," in *2012 International Conference on Computerized Healthcare*, Hong Kong: IEEE, 2012, pp. 134–139.

64. Z. Gu, R. Eils, M. Schlesner, and N. Ishaque, "EnrichedHeatmap: An R/ Bioconductor package for comprehensive visualization of genomic signal associations," *BMC Genomics*, vol. 19, p. 234. https://doi.org/10.1186/s12864-018-4625-x.

65. O. Rübel, G. H. Weber, S. V. Keränen, C. C. Fowlkes, C. L. L. Hendriks, L. Simirenko, N. Y. Shah, M. B. Eisen, M. D. Biggin, and H. Hagen, "PointCloudXplore: Visual analysis of 3D gene expression data using physical views and parallel coordinates," *EuroVis*, 2006, pp. 203–210.

66. J. Heinrich and D. Weiskopf, "State of the art of parallel coordinates," *Eurographics (State of the Art Reports)*, pp. 95–116, 2013.

67. P. Eades, "A heuristic for graph drawing," *Congressus Numerantium*, vol. 42, pp. 149–160, 1984.

68. T. M. J. Fruchterman and E. M. Reingold, "Graph drawing by force-directed placement," *Software: Practice and Experience*, vol. 21, pp. 1129–1164, 1991. https://doi.org/10.1002/spe.4380211102.

69. Z. Qu, C. W. Lau, Q. V. Nguyen, Y. Zhou, and D. R. Catchpoole, "Visual analytics of genomic and cancer data: A systematic review," *Cancer Informatics*, vol. 18, p. 1176935119835546, 2019. doi:10.1177/1176935119835546.

70. J. E. Venson, J. Berni, C. S. Maia, A. M. d. Silva, M. d'Ornelas, and A. Maciel, "Medical imaging VR: Can immersive 3D aid in diagnosis?," in *Proceedings of the 22nd ACM Conference on Virtual Reality Software and Technology*, Munich, 2016, pp. 349–350. https://doi.org/10.1145/2993369.2996333.

71. K. Dockx, E. M. Bekkers, V. Van den Bergh, P. Ginis, L. Rochester, J. M. Hausdorff, A. Mirelman, and A. Nieuwboer, "Virtual reality for rehabilitation in Parkinson's disease," *Cochrane Database of Systematic Reviews*, vol. 12, p. Cd010760, 2016. https://doi.org/10.1002/14651858.CD010760.pub2.

72. Q. V. Nguyen, Z. Qu, M. L. Huang, C. W. Lau, S. Simoff, and D. R. Catchpoole, "A mobile tool for interactive visualisation of genomics data," in *2018 9th International Conference on Information Technology in Medicine and Education (ITME)*, Hangzhou, 2018, pp. 688–697. ITME.

73. Z. Tang, C. Li, K. Zhang, M. Yang, and X. Hu, "GE-mini: a mobile APP for large-scale gene expression visualization," *Bioinformatics*, vol. 33, pp. 941–943, 2017. https://doi.org/10.1093/bioinformatics/btw775.

74. V. Liluashvili, S. Kalayci, E. Fluder, M. Wilson, A. Gabow, and Z. H. Gümüş, "iCAVE: an open source tool for visualizing biomolecular networks in 3D, stereoscopic 3D and immersive 3D," *GigaScience*, vol. 6, 2017. https://doi.org/10.1093/gigascience/gix054.

75. O. Legetth, J. Rodhe, J. Pålsson, M. Wallergård, S. Lang, and S. Soneji, "CellexalVR: A virtual reality platform for the exploration and analysis of single-cell gene expression data," *bioRxiv*, p. 329102, 2018.

76. A. Yang, Y. Yao, J. Li, and J. W. Ho, "Starmap: Immersive visualisation of single cell data using smartphone-enabled virtual reality," *bioRxiv*, p. 324855, 2018.

77. A. Maes, X. Martinez, K. Druart, B. Laurent, S. Guégan, C. H. Marchand, S. D. Lemaire, and M. Baaden, "MinOmics, an integrative and immersive tool for multi-omics analysis," *Journal of Integrative Bioinformatics*, vol. 15, 2018. https://doi.org/10.1515/jib-2018–0006.

78. J. F. Zhang, A. R. Paciorkowski, P. A. Craig, and F. Cui, "BioVR: A platform for virtual reality assisted biological data integration and visualization," *BMC Bioinformatics*, vol. 20, pp. 78–78, 2019. https://doi.org/10.1186/s12859–019–2666-z.

CHAPTER 9

Visualisation for Explainable Machine Learning in Biomedical Data Analysis

Zhonglin Qu, Simeon J. Simoff, Paul J. Kennedy, Daniel R. Catchpoole, and Quang Vinh Nguyen

9.1 INTRODUCTION

Large and complex data related to health status have been collected for the use of computers in biomedical and health-related fields to support data storage, security, and analysis [1]. Both clinical and non-clinical biomedical data are currently being collected for further analysis to find potential information inside. The massive amounts of biomedical data are analysed using statistical and other methods for new discoveries and advancement in the field of precision medicine [2, 3]. For example, vast amounts of mass cytometry single-cell data have been collected in a single experiment and can be analysed based on the arrangement of populations of cells such as cell type clusters [4–6]. This single-cell sequencing analysis can highlight somatic clonal structure, help track the formation of cell lineages, and provide insight into evolutionary processes acting on somatic mutations [7, 8].

There are some challenging themes in biomedical data analysis, such as quantifying the uncertainty of measurements and analysis results, scaling to higher dimensionalities, and varying levels of resolution [9]. New technologies can look at each of the individual cells. However, there is a limitation in real-time live tracking, disease prognosis analysis, and stem cell development [10]. For example, when mapping cell types and states for

DOI: 10.1201/9781003292357-9

their transcriptional relatedness, it is good to allow a choice of the level of resolution flexibly and to support the researcher in conveniently choosing the desired level of granularity with respect to the types and the states. Another challenge is determining subclone genotypes in more detail when integrating this with the spatial location. Handling sparsity in biomedical data is also challenging [11], for example, empty data for "drop-off" where a gene is expressed but not detected by the sequencing technology. A significant task in analysing high-dimensional biomedical data is to acceptable low-dimensional representations of the data that capture the salient biological signals and render the data more interpretable and amenable to further analyses [12]. Principal component analysis (PCA) is one of the standard matrix factorisation methods that can be applied to biomedical data such as in [13–15]. Comparing dimensionality reduction methods would help in exploring parameter spaces. Detailed benchmarking would help to establish when normalisation methods are derived from explicit models [2, 16]. Current analysis methods rely on dimensionality reduction, projection, and clustering to identify the subgroups of samples [17]. The lack of appropriate and available references and prevalent methods for identifying cell types has so far implied that only reference-free approaches were conceivable [18, 19].

Artificial intelligence (AI) and machine learning (ML) approaches have been used in various fields and have achieved outstanding success, including in the medical domain for biomedical data analysis [20–22]. ML algorithms are used for outcome classification, which is using one or more independent variables to determine an outcome, such as the prediction of stroke outcome [23] and estimation, prediction, and assistance in decision-making. The performance and efficiency in classifying multi-category outcomes of biomedical data accuracy of different ML models are calculated [24]. Some ML that is used for predicting the collective response of cancer patients to drugs has very high accuracy (>80%) [24]. Although computational decision-making methods are getting more and more accurate, it is often a struggle to move from pilot works to production due to the lack of trust in the AI or ML models from domain users [25]. Moreover, the General Data Protection Regulation (GDPR) has article 22 [26], "Automated Individual Decision-Making, Including Profiling", to set up the scope of the rights and obligations of automated decisions. The right of explanation is given to users to obtain an explanation of the AI or ML results and decision-making process [26]. There are more reasons for

ML explanation, such as trust, causality, transferability, informativeness, fair and ethical decision-making, accountability, adjustments, and proxy functionality [22].

ML explanation happens in different stages of the applications; some are built at the beginning of the model creation, and some are created after model creation. They also work on specific cases and ML algorithms, such as [27], to explain the decision tree model and decision-making process, [6] to explain UMAP with PCA methods, [28] to explain random forest classification ensembles, and [29] to explain neural networks. Visualisation techniques are used in these interpretations to empower the explanation process and increase domain users' trust. Some algorithms are linear and counted as "white boxes", such as PCA and decision trees, while some algorithms are non-linear and counted as "black boxes", such as uniform manifold approximation and projection (UMAP).

In this chapter, we discuss different visualisation methods to interpret supervised and unsupervised machine learning models in the biomedical data analysis domain. We present a case study for combining different interpretable machine learning methods to work on a complex biomedical data analysis. Some are for the supervised machine learning method random forest (RF), and some are for unsupervised machine learning methods such as UMAP.

9.2 INTERPRETABLE MACHINE LEARNING

There are two main ML streams: supervised ML and unsupervised ML.

Supervised ML is used for labelled data, and it aims to predict or classify a specific outcome of interest or target [30]. Supervised ML, such as logistic regression (LR), support vector machine (SVM), decision tree (DT), and random forest (RF), uses a labelled training dataset to train the underlying algorithm and then feeds the trained model on the unlabelled test dataset [31]. Supervised ML interpretation usually focuses on the model explanation, post-hoc black box explanation, and feature summary.

Unsupervised ML is used for unlabelled data to cluster and identify patterns in the dataset [32]. There are not many methods for directly explaining unsupervised ML, but some related methods are applied, for example, the methods to rank and select features before and after applying for unsupervised ML, such as a list of examples in the review of feature selection techniques in bioinformatics [33]. There are several methods for feature selection, including filter methods used to evaluate the relevance of each feature, wrapper methods used to evaluate the performance of different feature subsets, embedded methods used to integrate feature selection into the learning algorithm itself, and hybrid methods that combine different methods for improved performance. Some supervised ML techniques are also used in unsupervised interpretable ML, for example, using neural networks to explain the clusters [34], using a linear unsupervised method to explain the more complex non-linear unsupervised ML [6], and using LIME to interpret the cluster assignment decisions in the EXPLAIN-IT approach [35].

The trained ML model is presented in formulas as $\check{f}$ or $\check{f}(x)$. A row in the dataset consists of the feature values $x^{(i)}$, and the target outcome is y_i. The matrix with all features is called X and $x^{(i)}$ for a single instance. The vector of a single feature for all instances is x_j, and the value for the feature j and instance i is $x_j^{(i)}$. The target is usually called y or y_i. The model prediction is denoted by $\check{f}\left(x^{(i)}\right)$ or $\check{y}$ [20].

As shown in Figure 9.1, visualisation methods can show the supervised ML-trained model, decision path, and feature selection results. Visualisation for unsupervised ML can use brushing and linkable interactive plots to explain a black-box non-linear method with white-box linear methods, such as using principal component analysis to explain uniform manifold approximation and projection [36]. Heat-map visualisations can be used to show the classification results [35]. Bar charts can be used to show the ranked selected features [34]. Visualisation methods use various graphical representations to help users understand the inner working of the machine learning system and the decision process. Visualisation methods can be an effective way to make AI systems more transparent and accessible to users, providing a better understanding of the decision-making process and the factors that influence the AI's decisions.

Unsupervised interpretable machine learning is a subfield of machine learning that focuses on developing models that can understand and explain their own decision-making processes without the need for labelled data. This is achieved through the use of techniques such as feature selection, dimensionality reduction, and visualisation. Some popular unsupervised interpretable machine learning methods include principal component analysis [37], t-distributed stochastic neighbour embedding (t-SNE) [38], and autoencoders. The goal of unsupervised interpretable machine learning is to create models that are both accurate and transparent, making it easier for humans to understand and trust the decisions made by the

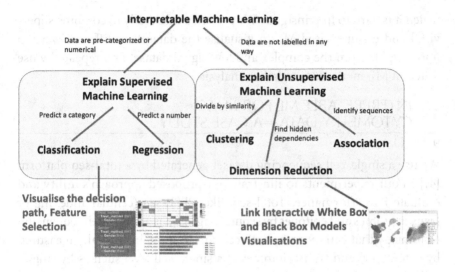

FIGURE 9.1 Interpretable machine learning methods for supervised and unsupervised machine learning methods. Visualisation methods can show the supervised ML-trained model, decision path, and feature selection results. Unsupervised ML visualisation can use brushing and linkable interactive plots to explain a black-box non-linear method with white-box linear methods.

model. The unsupervised ML method dimensionality reduction (DR) uses machine learning techniques to transform high-dimensional data into meaningful low-dimensional data with minimal information loss before proceeding with the analysis. The reduced dimension space must have correspondence to the intrinsic data dimensionality [39]. DR is frequently used for data compression, exploration, and visualisation. Low-dimensional data representations remove noise but retain the signal of interest to understand hidden structures and patterns [40]. There are many DR methods, such as linear method principal component analysis, non-linear method t-distributed stochastic neighbour embedding (t-SNE) and uniform manifold approximation and projection [36]. PCA is a good choice if the underlying structure of a dataset is known to be relatively linear. t-SNE is the proper choice for a non-linear structured dataset, but it is too slow when applied to large datasets. In contrast, UMAP [36] is a new method, and it is claimed to be more scalable and more accurate than t-SNE [38].

Some biomedical data, such as omics single-cell data, have sample level labels and multiple dimensions with only values of different numbers, for which it is hard to find insights. We present a case study to combine supervised and unsupervised ML to visualise the dataset in different ways to find insights from the complex and low-signal dataset and repeatedly use different ML methods for further analysis.

9.3 INTERPRETABLE ML FOR MASS CYTOMETRY DATA—A CASE STUDY

9.3.1 Data

We use a single-cell sequencing dataset generated by a total-seq platform [41] in our experiments to illustrate our proposed approach's utility and evaluate its performance. Total-seq, like CITE-seq (cellular indexing of transcriptomes and epitopes by sequencing [42]), is a single-cell sequencing technology that can measure both cell surface proteins (usually measured by cytometry) and transcriptomes at a single-cell level such as by single-cell RNA sequencing (scRNA-seq). Therefore, the number of dimensions of a total-seq dataset can be much higher than flow cytometry or RNA sequencing data.

The dataset has 12 deidentified human PBMC samples by combining four treatment/stimulation conditions and three titration levels. The four treatments include Control (control PBMC: no stimulation or cultured overnight), IFNgTNFa (IFN-gamma and TNF alpha stimulation), IL2 (IL2 stimulation), and ON (Cultured Overnight). The three titration levels are 0.25×, 1×, and 4×. For each comparison, we merged the 12 samples by concatenation, resulting in a table with 24,410 rows and 202 columns. Each row corresponds to a single cell with quantitative measurements of the surface protein expressions (e.g., CD3, CD19 etc.), and each column name is a molecule marker. The missing values in the dataset are replaced with zero.

9.3.2 Methods

We use two more interpretable ML algorithms, PCA, and SHapley Additive exPlanations (SHAP) [43], on random forest (RF) [44] to explain a more complex method that was more effective in identifying sub-populations in single-cell sequencing datasets, uniform manifold approximation, and projection [36]. Challenges in mass cytometry single-cell data analysis have been addressed, such as interactively determining subclone genotypes in more detail in spatial location and real-time tracking the subsets of single cell groups. The combination of the three methods, PCA, UMAP, and RF, can also find the most important markers for further investigation of the diseases. This analysis aims to find insights in the data and explain the complex machine learning method for domain users to gain their trust to take actions based on the computational results.

As shown in Figure 9.2, we combined supervised and unsupervised ML visualisations for a biomedical data analysis. Unsupervised ML PCA and UMAP are used to cluster similar groups and extract the important features, and the supervised ML random forest is used to rank the features before the unsupervised ML and can also be used after the unsupervised ML for making a prediction. There are two cycles in this framework: one is to extract rules, and the other is to use the rules and make decisions. The whole dataset was processed with two unsupervised ML methods, UMAP and PCA. Linkable and interactive scatter plots were generated. As the dataset had sample-level labels, we applied the supervised ML random forest to it and run the explainable ML model SHAP on it. SHAP was a model-agnostic framework for interpreting predictions, based on estimating the contribution of each feature for a particular prediction [43]. SHAP was created based on the principles from the cooperative game theory called coalitional games [45]. Shapley values are used in game theory to fairly distribute surplus across a coalition of players [46]. In the SHAP model, input features and Shapley values replaced players to show the contribution to a given predicted result. In genomic studies, SHAP has been used

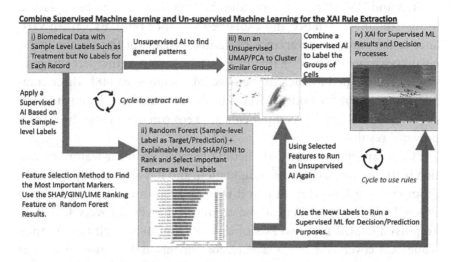

FIGURE 9.2 Combined supervised and unsupervised ML visualisations for a biomedical data analysis.

to identify biomarkers [21]. For example, DeepSHAP [47] was a model used to explain the predictions of a deep neural network. The purpose of this step was to rank all the features and find the most important ones to run the unsupervised ML again for better accuracy. Another purpose was to use the most important features as the targeted labels to run the supervised ML again for a prediction or a decision. After the most important features were extracted, these features could become new labels of the data to run a supervised ML for decision-making purposes.

9.3.3 Results

We visualised the three DR methods, UMAP, t-SNE, and PCA, in 3D and 2D spaces and calculated the running time, as shown in Figure 9.3 and Table 9.1 respectively. We compare the three methods and choose two of them to apply to the biomedical dataset based on the computational cost and the clustering abilities. As shown in Table 9.1, UMAP and t-SNE have better clustering abilities than PCA, as shown in each scatter plot. T-SNE has highest computational cost (392 seconds), followed by UMAP (40 seconds), and PCA is the fastest one (0.23 seconds). Table 9.1 explains the variance ratio of the three DR methods: UMAP, t-SNE, and PCA. UMAP and t-SNE can distinguish clusters better than PCA. T-SNE used the most time, 392 seconds, and PCA is the fastest one at 0.23 seconds. UMAP used 40 seconds, which is faster than t-SNE.

PCA and UMAP components and their significance can be explained using explained variance and explained variance ratio. Explained variance is the amount of variance explained by each of the selected principal components (PCs). Explained variance ratio is the percentage of variance explained by each of the selected components [48]. Three components are kept for both UMAP and PCA methods and shown in bar charts at first. Then five components are kept comparing the three components' results.

PCA is an interpretable ML method because its linear feature extraction is straightforward in the computation, and it is analytically traceable. From Figure 9.4, we can see that if we only keep three PCs, the first two PCs of UMAP cover 69% of all the variance, while PCA covers 82%. If we keep five PCs, the first two PCs of UMAP cover 48% of all the variance, while PCA covers 68%. PCA is better for dimension deduction, as it keeps more values of all attributes. Keeping fewer PCs makes the first two PCs cover more variances.

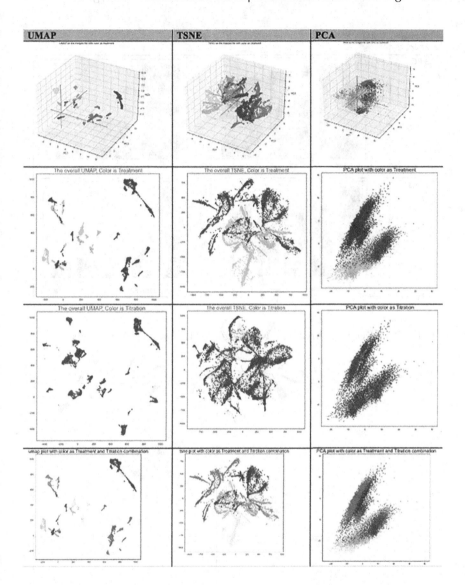

FIGURE 9.3 The UMAP, TSNE, and PCA projection and clustering results for the same dataset. Explained variance ratio of the three DR methods: UMAP, t-SNE, and PCA. UMAP and t-SNE can distinguished clusters better than PCA.

TABLE 9.1 The Total Processed Time for Each Method for the Same Dataset

	UMAP	TSNE	PCA
Total Processed Time (seconds)	40.28	393.00	0.24

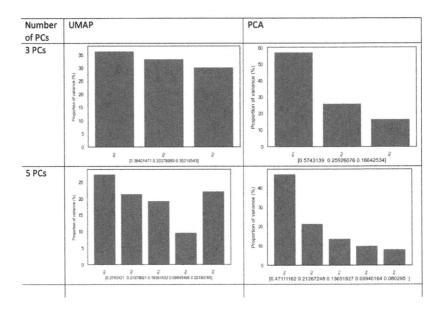

FIGURE 9.4   Keeping three and five PCs for UMAP and PCA methods.

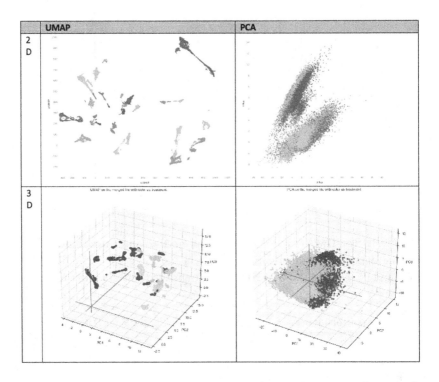

FIGURE 9.5   Comparing 2D and 3D UMAP and PCA. The UMAP plots can cluster similar cells better than the PCA plots.

We then plot the UMAP and PCA in 2D and 3D space, as shown in Figure 9.5. From the observations and comparisons, UMAP plots can cluster the similar cells better than PCA plots. There is not much difference between 2D and 3D plots. It is easier to add interactions to the 2D plots because of the existing software. So, we choose 2D to add interactions and link the PCA and UMAP plots together. We show the interactive linkable 2D plots in Figures 9.6 and 9.7. Figure 9.6 shows the PCA and UMAP results in one dashboard and can be filtered with the same group labels in the legend. Figure 9.7 shows a group label to highlight one subgroup, IFNgTNFa, 1x, in both UMAP and PCA plots.

As the data have labels Treatment and Titration, we can also run a supervised machine learning model random forest. The explainable model SHAP is used on top of the random forest to find the important markers. We then plot the most important 20 markers as bar charts. Then PCA and UMAP are run again based on the seven most important markers. Interactive scatter plot visualisations with brushing and linked techniques [49] are developed for users to drill down their interesting features. The random forest algorithm picks random records from the dataset and builds a decision tree with these records, then repeats these two steps to build multiple decision trees. In this case, we build a group of decision

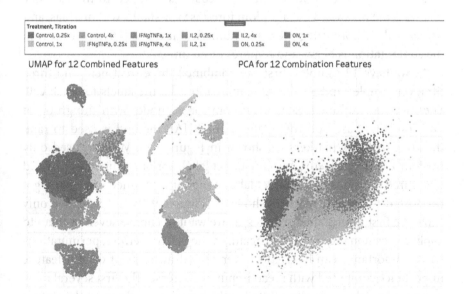

FIGURE 9.6 Linking UMAP and PCA plots with the same filter groups with the same colours. The clustering patterns are similar between UMAP and PCA.

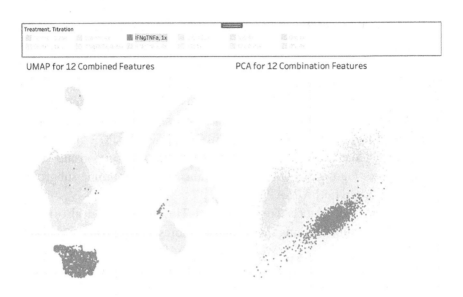

FIGURE 9.7 Highlighting one group, IFNgTNFa, 1x, in both UMAP and PCA plots. The same groups of cells are clustered most together; only a small portion of cells overlap other cells.

trees and then use SHAP to calculate the average of all the values predicted by all the trees in the forest. The new record is assigned to the category that wins the majority vote. Random forest is very stable, without bias, and works well for both categorical and numerical features [50, 51]. However, the computation is heavy and requires more time.

As we have 12 samples, first, we combined three treatment and three titration samples and let the 12 combinations be the labels for each cell. Then we trained and created a random forest model with the group of decision trees based on these labels. The SHAP method is used to rank the 202 attributes/markers, as shown in Figure 9.8a. We also used only the four treatment methods as the target labels for one trained model and only three titrations as the target labels for another trained model and got the sorted important markers shown in Figures 9.8b and 9.8c. We only show the first important attributes, as we want to choose seven of them to apply dimensionality reduction again. In the SHAP method, permutation-based importance can be used to overcome drawbacks of default feature importance computed with mean impurity decrease. The first several most important markers are also plotted with more details, showing the feature value.

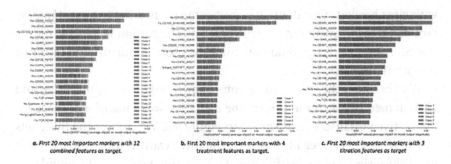

a. First 20 most important markers with 12 combined features as target.   *b. First 20 most important markers with 4 treatment features as target.*   *c. First 20 most important markers with 3 titration features as target*

FIGURE 9.8   Using SHAP on top of the random forest method and labels as targets to rank all the markers and show the first important 20 markers.

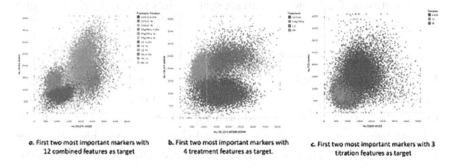

a. First two most important markers with 12 combined features as target   *b. First two most important markers with 4 treatment features as target.*   *c. First two most important markers with 3 titration features as target*

FIGURE 9.9   Plotting the first two important markers after ranking all the markers with SHAP. All three scatter plots show clear boundaries where the selected markers are the most important features.

The accuracy with the combined features as the target is 97.5%. The accuracy with the treatment features as the target is 98.7%. The accuracy with the titration features as the target is 99.0%.

To verify the SHAP results, we used the results to plot the first two important features with scatter plot visualisations, as shown in Figure 9.9. Figure 9.9a shows the first two important markers with 12 combined features as the target, coloured with 12 combined features. Figure 9.9b shows the first two important markers with four treatment features as the target, coloured with the four treatments. Figure 9.9c illustrates the first two most important markers with three titration features as the target, coloured with three titrations. We can see the three scatter plots all have clear boundaries based on the target colours in Figure 9.9. The figure indicates that the first two important markers can separate well the sub-populations with clear borders. Our domain expert confirms that the two most important markers for treatment are true based on the current facts. This means that SHAP for ranking could potentially be useful in identifying the most important markers.

We then use the seven most important markers to apply PCA and UMAP methods again to project the data to a two-dimensional space for interactive visualisation, as shown in Figure 9.6. We can see the three sets of UMAP and PCA results based on the three trained RF models all have good clustering and projection based on the target colours. We found that the three UMAP and PCA visualisations have good clustering bounders. The plotted visualisations are interactive; we can drill down each group of samples to the raw data. For example, we select Treatment as Control and Titration as 0.25, and then all six scatter plots will highlight the same group of cells.

9.4 CONCLUSION AND FUTURE WORK

In this chapter, we used a linear and more interpretable method, PCA, to explain a new and complex non-linear projection method, UMAP. An explainable model, SHAP, is used on a supervised AI model random forest to optimise the input data for PCA and UMAP. We provide interactive PCA and UMAP scatter plots for the processed data in the former computational analyses. The linking and brushing interactions can help users drill down the subsets of each sample and direct to go to the raw data. We find that the outcomes from the UMAP and PCA methods have some similar clustering and projection patterns, which leads to a hypothesis that we can use the interpretable PCA to explain UMAP. As the dataset has the sample level labels Treatment and Titration, we can also use the supervised AI model random forest and an explainable model, SHAP, to optimise the input data for the PCA and UMAP methods. The purpose of using SHAP on random forest is to rank all the markers so that the most important markers can be identified for UMAP and PCA methods. This step can improve the accuracy of the dimensionality reduction. The results are then used to apply back to UMAP and PCA to get more accurate projection and clustering visualisations.

The new sets of interactive UMAP and PCA visualisations are also interactive. Users can highlight any sub-group of the cell samples in both UMAP and PCA to check the similarity and differences. We believe the analysis results and the result comparisons can help domain users trust the new machine learning method, UMAP, based on the results of the familiar method, PCA. The outputs with supporting interactive visualisation can also help domain users do further investigation and assist in decision-making.

Next we will work more on the comparisons among the different dimensionality reduction methods and find meaningful features to help elucidate novel biomarkers in the continuum of cells. The work could potentially help domain users better understand the new machine learning models and improve their trust in the models. After the most important features are identified with the dimensionality reduction methods, the features can be used as new targeted labels and be applied to a new supervised ML method, such as RF or a neural network, for a new prediction or a new output to help decision-making. The new extracted features work as new supervised ML labels.

REFERENCES

1. Zubairu, B., Security Risks of Biomedical Data Processing in Cloud Computing Environment, in Cloud Security: Concepts, Methodologies, Tools, and Applications. 2019, IGI Global. pp. 1748–1768.
2. Mirza, B., et al., Machine Learning and Integrative Analysis of Biomedical Big Data. Genes, 2019. 10(2): p. 87.
3. Lau, C.W., et al., Virtual Reality for the Observation of Oncology Models (VROOM): Immersive Analytics for Oncology Patient Cohorts. Scientific Reports, 2022. 12(1): p. 11337.
4. Spitzer, Matthew H. and Garry P. Nolan, Mass Cytometry: Single Cells, Many Features. Cell, 2016. 165(4): pp. 780–791.
5. Tegegne, Y., et al. Parallel Nonlinear Dimensionality Reduction Using GPU Acceleration. 2021, Springer.
6. Qu, Z., et al. Enhancing Understandability of Omics Data with SHAP, Embedding Projections and Interactive Visualisations. in Australasian Conference on Data Mining. 2022, Springer.
7. Francis, J.M., et al., EGFR Variant Heterogeneity in Glioblastoma Resolved through Single-Nucleus Sequencing. Cancer Discover, 2014. 4(8): pp. 956–971.
8. Lawson, D.A., et al., Tumour Heterogeneity and Metastasis at Single-cell Resolution. Nature Cell Biology, 2018. 20(12): pp. 1349–1360.
9. Lähnemann, D., et al., Eleven Grand Challenges in single-cell data science. Genome Biology, 2020. 21(1): pp. 31–35.
10. Wong, K.-C., Big Data Challenges in Genome Informatics. Biophysical Reviews, 2018. 11.
11. Chi, W. and M. Deng, Sparsity-Penalized Stacked Denoising Autoencoders for Imputing Single-Cell RNA-Seq Data. Genes, 2020. 11(5): p. 532.
12. Pierson, E. and C. Yau, ZIFA: Dimensionality Reduction for Zero-inflated Single-cell Gene Expression Analysis. Genome Biology, 2015. 16(1): pp. 241–241.

13. Tsuyuzaki, K., et al., Benchmarking Principal Component Analysis for Large-scale Single-cell RNA-sequencing. Genome Biology, 2020. **21**(1): pp. 1–17.

14. Qi, R., et al., Clustering and Classification Methods for Single-cell RNA-sequencing Data. Briefings in Bioinformatics, 2020. **21**(4): pp. 1196–1208.

15. Dou, M., et al., High-throughput Single Cell Proteomics Enabled by Multiplex Isobaric Labeling in a Nanodroplet Sample Preparation Platform. Analytical Chemistry, 2019. **91**(20): pp. 13119–13127.

16. Heaton, H., et al., Souporcell: Robust Clustering of Single-cell RNA-seq Data by Genotype without Reference Genotypes. Nature Methods, 2020. **17**(6): pp. 615–620.

17. Yang, Y., et al., SAFE-clustering: Single-cell Aggregated (from Ensemble) Clustering for Single-cell RNA-seq Data. Bioinformatics, 2019. **35**(8): pp. 1269–1277.

18. Aran, D., et al., Reference-based Analysis of Lung Single-cell Sequencing Reveals A Transitional Profibrotic Macrophage. Nature Immunology, 2019. **20**(2): pp. 163–172.

19. Wang, X., et al., Bulk Tissue Cell Type Deconvolution with Multi-subject Single-cell Expression Reference. Nature Communications, 2019. **10**(1): pp. 1–9.

20. Molnar, C., Interpretable Machine Learning. 2020, Lulu.

21. Watson, D., Interpretable Machine Learning for Genomics. Human Genetics, 2021. **141**: pp. 1499–1513.

22. Burkart, N. and M.F. Huber, A Survey on the Explainability of Supervised Machine Learning. Journal of Artificial Intelligence Research, 2021. **70**: pp. 245–317.

23. Heo, T.S., et al., Prediction of Stroke Outcome Using Natural Language Processing-based Machine Learning of Radiology Report of Brain MRI. Journal of Personalized Medicine, 2020. **10**(4): p. 286.

24. Deng, F., et al., Performance and Efficiency of Machine Learning Algorithms for Analyzing Rectangular Biomedical Data. Laboratory Investigation, 2021. **101**(4): pp. 430–441.

25. Cruz, J.A. and D.S. Wishart, Applications of Machine Learning in Cancer Prediction and Prognosis. Cancer Informatics, 2006. **2**: p. 11769351 0600200030.

26. GDPR. Automated Individual Decision-making, Including Profiling. General Data Protection Regulation (GDPR) 2022 [cited 2022]; Available from: https://gdpr-info.eu/art-22-gdpr/.

27. Qu, Z., et al., Using Visualization to Illustrate Machine Learning Models for Genomic Data. 2019, ACM.

28. Neto, M.P. and F.V. Paulovich, Explainable Matrix-visualization for Global and Local Interpretability of Random Forest Classification Ensembles. IEEE Transactions on Visualization and Computer Graphics, 2020. **27**(2): pp. 1427–1437.

29. Wang, Z.J., et al., CNN Explainer: Learning Convolutional Neural Networks with Interactive Visualization. IEEE Transactions on Visualization and Computer Graphics, 2020. **27**(2): pp. 1396–1406.

30. Jiang, T., J.L. Gradus, and A.J. Rosellini, Supervised Machine Learning: A Brief Primer. Behavior Therapy, 2020. **51**(5): pp. 675–687.
31. Uddin, S., et al., Comparing Different Supervised Machine Learning Algorithms for Disease Prediction. BMC Medical Informatics and Decision Making, 2019. **19**(1): p. 281.
32. Li, N., M. Shepperd, and Y. Guo, A systematic Review of Unsupervised Learning Techniques for Software Defect Prediction. Information and Software Technology, 2020. **122**: p. 106287.
33. Saeys, Y., I. Inza, and P. Larrañaga, A Review of Feature Selection Techniques in Bioinformatics. Bioinformatics, 2007. **23**(19): pp. 2507–2517.
34. Kauffmann, J., et al., From Clustering to Cluster Explanations via Neural Networks. IEEE Transactions on Neural Networks and Learning Systems, 2022: pp. 1–15.
35. Morichetta, A., P. Casas, and M. Mellia. EXPLAIN-IT: Towards Explainable AI for Unsupervised Network Traffic Analysis. 2020, Cornell University Library. arXiv.org.
36. Becht, E., et al., Dimensionality Reduction for Visualizing Single-cell Data Using UMAP. Nature Biotechnology, 2018. **37**(1): pp. 38–44.
37. Hosoya, H. and A. Hyvärinen, Learning Visual Spatial Pooling by Strong PCA Dimension Reduction. Neural Computation, 2016. **28**(7): p. 1249.
38. Konstorum, A., et al., Comparative Analysis of Linear and Nonlinear Dimension Reduction Techniques on Mass Cytometry Data. bioRxiv, 2018: p. 273862.
39. Sumithra, V.S. and S. Subu, A Review of Various Linear and Non Linear Dimensionality Reduction Techniques. International Journal of Computer Science and Information Technologies, 2015. **6**(3).
40. Nguyen, L.H. and S. Holmes, Ten Quick Tips for Effective Dimensionality Reduction. PLoS Computational Biology, 2019. **15**(6): p. e1006907.
41. BioLegend. Comprehensive Solutions for Single-Cell and Bulk Multiomics. 2021 [cited 2021]; Available from: www.biolegend.com/en-us/totalseq?gcli d=CjwKCAjwx8iIBhBwEiwA2quaq0V-IkCRsY9UZ6G1Lop5Tfd0dl1m_ YF-_fyd-1Hgz5fUvpEvevRpcRoCIjUQAvD_BwE.
42. Stoeckius, M., et al., Simultaneous Epitope and Transcriptome Measurement in Single Cells. Nature Methods, 2017. **14**(9): pp. 865–868.
43. Lundberg, S.M. and S.-I. Lee, A Unified Approach to Interpreting Model Predictions, in Proceedings of the 31st International Conference on Neural Information Processing Systems. 2017, Curran Associates Inc.: Long Beach, CA, pp. 4768–4777.
44. Dimitriadis, S. and D. Liparas, How Random is the Random Forest? Random Forest Algorithm on the Service of Structural Imaging Biomarkers for Alzheimer's Disease: From Alzheimer's Disease Neuroimaging Initiative (ADNI) Database. Neural Regeneration Research, 2018. **13**(6): pp. 962–970.
45. Osborne, M.J., A Course in Game Theory, ed. A. Rubinstein. 2006, MIT Press.
46. Shapley, L.S., H. Kuhn, and A. Tucker, Contributions to the Theory of Games. Annals of Mathematics studies, 1953. **28**(2): pp. 307–317.
47. Pernando, Z.T., J. Singh, and A. Anand. A study on the Interpretability of Neural Retrieval Models using Deep SHAP, in Proceedings of the 42nd

International ACM SIGIR Conference on Research and Development in Information Retrieval, ACM, 2019, pp. 1005–1008.

48. Lindgren, I. Dealing with Highly Dimensional Data using Principal Component Analysis (PCA). Towards Data Science 2020 [cited 2020]; Available from: https://towardsdatascience.com/dealing-with-highly-dimensional-data-using-principal-component-analysis-pca-fea1ca817fe6.

49. Radoš, S., et al., Towards Quantitative Visual Analytics with Structured Brushing and Linked Statistics. Computer Graphics Forum, 2016. **35**(3): pp. 251–260.

50. Arora, N. and P.D. Kaur, A Bolasso Based Consistent Feature Selection Enabled Random Forest Classification Algorithm: An Application to Credit Risk Assessment. Applied Soft Computing, 2020. **86**: p. 105936.

51. Aria, M., C. Cuccurullo, and A. Gnasso, A comparison Among Interpretative Proposals for Random Forests. Machine Learning with Applications, 2021. **6**: p. 100094.

CHAPTER 10

Visual Communication and Trust in the Health Domain

Quang Vinh Nguyen, Paul J. Kennedy, Simeon J. Simoff, and Daniel R. Catchpoole

10.1 INTRODUCTION

Effective and trustful communication of analytical and exploration results is crucial in the decision-making process [1]. Complex visualisation methods are useful for analysts who normally spend adequate time for training and deeply exploring biomedical data. However, it is often a challenge for high-level decision makers (such as clinicians or executive managers) and public readers who might not be able to perceive well the complex visualisations. Thus, post-edition and selection of final presentations to highlight the discovery or story through simplified and enhanced visualisations are often essential steps in biomedical research [2]. By using well-known graphical representations in the domain, such as diagrammatic visualisations and domain visual metaphors, the final views could lead to superior communications to executive decision-makers and public users.

Figure 10.1 shows an example of a diagrammatic visualisation of logistic data at Port Botany, Sydney, Australia, resulting from the study in [3]. By using the domain visual metaphors and icons, the figure clearly presents the performance and productivity indicators of trucks and slots at the ports at a particular time.

Steering and refining machine learning models with domain knowledge are not trivial tasks and may accumulate bias. There is widespread concern

DOI: 10.1201/9781003292357-10

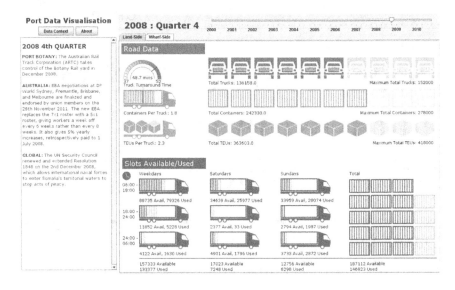

FIGURE 10.1 An example of diagrammatic visualisation of the performance of trucks and slots at a particular time.

about trust in data and computational methods due to cultural history, data, omission, bias certainty, and precision [4]. The trust issue of computational analytics outcomes is always an obstacle in data analytics, especially in conservative domains, such as the health and biomedical fields. Trust includes accuracy (correctness or freedom from mistakes), precision (exactness or degree of refinement), and trustworthiness (dependability or the confidence of the users) [5]. In terms of data analytics, trustworthiness is the property of the data, visualisation, computational model, communication, or process that can lead the users to trust it. Trust is normally associated with the transparency of the information and disclosure of underlying data or decisions, usually including interaction to improve trustworthiness. Trust is normally derived from users' assessment and evaluation of a visualisation, a model, a process, or an output.

Interpretable machine learning, or in a broader term, explainable artificial intelligence (XAI), has been gradually studied and applied to explain the "black boxes" of machine learning models or complex computational analytics processes, such as those comprehensively reviewed in [1, 6]. The explanations can be classified into four main areas [7]:

- *Explain to justify*—show how the explanation can be used to illustrate the underlying model to improve the justification.

- *Explain to control*—use the explanation for enhancing the transparency of a model or a function for reducing bugs or flaws.

- *Explain to improve*—use the explanation to improve the accuracy and efficiency of the models.

- *Explain to discover*—support the extraction of insight and discovery of patterns.

10.2 TRUST IN HEALTH DATA-DRIVEN SCIENCE

Trust is one of the greatest challenges for real-life computational analytics and applications and is crucial to support users in making sense of the information and being aware of uncertainties in the data [8, 9]. It is shown that there is an association between trust and outcomes in the health domain [10]. For example, patients are more satisfied with the provided treatment or diagnosis when they gain more trust in healthcare professionals.

However, there are many unanswered questions and challenges in the field. For example, if a user is not aware of the uncertainties and trust issues in a machine learning model, how do we ensure that she will not have a wrong assumption about the model; or that she is not deceived by false or unclear results; or what is the problem with the trustworthiness of the model? [5] Domain experts might not be likely to use a computational model if they do not understand how the model works, especially in medical data analytics [11]. In addition, non-expert and novice users in analytics, such as clinicians, also want to gain trust in the models when making a decision on treatments and diagnoses.

Health domain experts and practitioners usually use visualisation techniques to enhance trust in machine learning models thanks to their effectiveness in improving the understanding, interpretability, and explainability of the complexity of machine learning models [5, 12]. Biologists and doctors can be interested in comparing data structures and receiving guidance on the focus area in visualisation.

High-cognitive people are more influenced by the quality of work, which is an important factor leading to different trust perceptions between domain experts and casual ones. Also, a critical decision in the health domain also affects a decision where users care more about the trustfulness of a method or an output [8]. Healthcare professionals, such as clinicians, normally endure more scepticism and doubts about AI-based systems due to their prior experiences as well as the conservative and critical decision-making nature of the field [13]. Therefore, it is essential to provide targeted communication with effective design and training for such users in the health domain.

However, clinical and health data are very large and complex, which also brings many challenges and opportunities. For example, clinicians try to make sense of the data by combining the data from different systems, administrators make decisions based on grounded data, researchers try to understand data via exploration, and patients try to make sense of their own medical data [14]. However, large amounts of information also increase the overload, where the number of variables can easily surpass human capacity [15]. This issue leads to users ignoring, overlooking, or misinterpreting crucial information. There have been widespread issues in the healthcare domain that can lead to incorrect interpretations of data, wrong diagnoses, and missed warning signs of impending changes to patient conditions [14].

Visual analytics and interactive visualisation can help to improve the transparency of the analysis and obtain insights from large amounts of clinical data. Yet visualisation might lead to a compromise on trust, and improving trustworthiness in machine learning with visualisation is also related to improving trust for visualisation [16]. There is a need to develop further guidelines and best practices in heath data analytics.

10.3 ANALYTICAL PROCESSES AND TRUST LEVELS

Trust is linked with computational analytics, which are all connected to evaluation and user expectation via visualisation and interaction. Trust could be classified into six levels following the analytical processes, as shown in Figure 10.2.

- **Trust in raw data (trust level 1)**—refers to the source's reliability and the transparency of the data collection process to avoid the fear of "garbage in, garbage out" in critical and precise health data. By visualising this process and providing the ability to access and manipulate the original data, we can improve the acceptability of the quality and behaviour of the data by users [17].

- **Trust in processed data (trust level 2)**—focuses on whether the pre-processed data are reliable and clean, such as filtering out unfitting instances or borderline case data, ensuring minimal bias in the data.

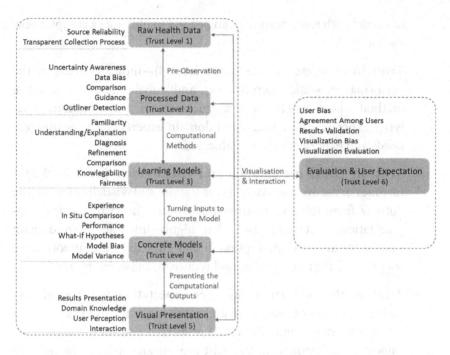

FIGURE 10.2 The trust levels for analytical processes of health data, adapted from [5].

Visualisation is essential for comparing different structures [18]; providing guidance and recommendations on new labels in unlabelled data scenarios; or managing data by adding, removing, and merging data [19]. For example, by viewing and detecting extreme values in a meaningful way, we can boost overall trust, and it is a useful way to influent results.

- **Trust in learning methods and algorithms (trust level 3)**—shows the familiarity of the use of visualisation to support a user to get familiar with and understand machine learning methods. For example, the user needs to gain knowledge of a machine learning model and its behaviour or diagnose the reasons for unsuccessful convergence or failure to achieve a satisfactory performance. Such guidance for both expert and novice users can boost the performance, transparency, and quality of machine learning models through the refinement and comparison of different algorithms. A simpler and more interpretable model, such as a rule-based model, linear model, or model with fewer features, can be used to illustrate a complex one, such as [12].

• **Trust in concrete models (trust level 4)**—indicates trust in the performance, static interpretation, and a dynamic and interactive method where experience is a crucial factor. Computational analytics experts, novice users, and domain experts can have different needs and experiences in visualisations.

• **Trust in visual presentation and visualisation (trust level 5)**—includes trust in the visual presentation and visualisation of the outputs from the computational analytics. The visual design, representation, and interaction that highly integrate with domain knowledge and user perception design guidelines are important to supplement the trust process and reduce visualisation bias.

• **Trust in the evaluation and user expectation (trust level 6)**—includes choices of evaluation and results validations in the visualisation and interaction. The visual properties and representation are important to supplement the trust process and reduce visualisation bias. Validation uses a visualisation tool to indicate if a computational model or data can be trusted or meet the user's expectations. Unfortunately, there is still a lack of studies on user bias to understand the cognitive bias of their involvement in decision-making from automated analysis models.

10.4 TRUST ISSUES IN COMPUTATIONAL ANALYTICS AND VISUALISATION

Trust is dynamic based on the user's accumulated experience, interaction, case scenario, and problem awareness on a method or a model. The trust issue also depends on the user's background, expertise, personality, and social environment [20]. Computational analytic models and methods might not be trusted by end users due to their complexity and un-interpretability, or might be a so-called black box, so interactive visualisation is essential to bridge the gaps, foster trust in learning and analytical models, and increase the awareness of interdisciplinary users.

Familiarity with a visualisation method can increase trust and readability, while novel visualisation methods might not be well perceived by the users [21]. Without prior knowledge or experience in the models or the process, other trust processes will likely be activated. Thus, users with prior positive experiences in visualisation, statistical, and computational analyses will likely gain more trust in new outcomes and information [22]. In addition, poorly designed visualisations can reduce perception and increase cognitive overhead and processing complexity. The lack of clarity can confuse users and raise doubts about accuracy and certainty. For example, the misalignment of a visualisation and descriptive text could affect understanding.

Trust in information visualisation is multifaceted [23] and tightly connects to the transparency of the communication perceived by the users [24]. Unfortunately, there has been a lack of empirical studies on uncertainty and trust. Users with low prior knowledge of statistics, computational analytics, and visualisation may have a higher distrust of a method [8]. Users normally perceive the actual data as the most credible and the processed data as less so, which is especially important for highly crucial health domains. Thus, showing more underlying and original data can improve the trust of the users [17].

In addition, improvement in transparency can reduce speculation, mistrust of presented data, and mistrust in the reporting data [25]. When showing more information with visualisation, the uncertainty can increase trust [26]. However, having too much visual information might also increase confusion, which can negatively impact the accuracy of interpretations due to cognitive overload.

Although studies have been carried out on trust, such as those discussed in [4, 5, 8, 10], more research for understanding the long-term effects of trust is still required, especially in information visualisation [27]. Good visualisation can assist users to gain better insight into the trustworthiness of a method, especially for novices and casual users. When a user puts trust in a visualisation, what are the trust cues in a design, or how the user can perceive trust in a visualisation? [8]

There is still a lack of workable theory on how human–computer interaction and visualisation can build trust between the creators and the end users. Further studies are required to gain a holistic understanding of trustworthiness, fairness, interpretability, accountability, and other factors of AI [13]. The design choice of visualisation can also influent trust in a method, a model, a process, or an output. However, trust cannot be the only indication of successful interpretation. Visualisation methods should balance performance and trust [28].

10.5 MODELS AND METHODS FOR INTERPRETABILITY AND TRUST

For biomedical data analytics, visualisations are usually used to visually explain the analytics models and the predictive results in meaningful ways so that they can be understood and interpreted by the users, such as in [29]. However, it is challenging to understand how visualisation can boost a machine learning and deep learning model's trustworthiness. Numeric and mixed explanations are commonly used for measuring input variables and quantitative metrics of such complex biomedical data.

Convolutional neural networks (CNNs) are often the first step to provide a preliminary explanation to a user for black-box models. Specialised and targeted CNN models might show the analysis of insights that are retrieved from deep neural network models [30]. Recent works also foster awareness of the usefulness of having an interpretable machine learning model where explainability and interpretability are among the key factors for trustworthiness [31].

Explainable AI methods might integrate domain knowledge or simpler methods to explain complex models. AxiSketcher [32] includes domain knowledge on an interactive visualisation of t-SNE projection [33] for better comparison of clusters and identification of problematic cases. iFores [34] uses visualisation to show aggregated views with decision paths in random forest models for a better understanding of the decision paths of the algorithm. Recent work [12] uses the linear projection method principal component analysis (PCA) with interactive visualisation to explain the complex non-linear project method UMAP [35]. The authors also use SHapley Additive exPlanations (SHAP) [36] and random forest (RF) to select the significant features in the omics data.

SHAP [36] and local interpretable model-agnostic explanations (LIME) [37] are two popular methods that are commonly used for numeric and mixed explanations, respectively. LIME is a prescribed method for local interpretability used to explain the behaviours of the classifiers in terms of interpretable representations [37]. SHAP is another tool that can visualise the outputs of machine learning models by computing the contribution of each feature to the prediction, thus making the outputs and predictions more explainable [36]. Both methods have gradually gained attention in the biomedical data analytics community, such as in recent works [38–42].

10.6 CONCLUSION

This chapter explains the visual communication and trust aspects in health data-driven science. We present the association of the analytical processes and the corresponding trust levels, together with the evaluation and user expectation via interactive visualisation. The trust issues in current computational analytics and visualisation are also discussed in the chapter. Finally, the chapter briefly shows models and methods that can support improvement in interpretability and trust in the models, methods, and visualisations.

REFERENCES

1. G. Vilone and L. Longo, "Explainable Artificial Intelligence: A Systematic Review," https://arxiv.org/abs/2006.00093, 2020.
2. S. I. O'Donoghue, B. F. Baldi, S. J. Clark, A. E. Darling, J. M. Hogan, S. Kaur, L. Maier-Hein, D. J. McCarthy, W. J. Moore, E. Stenau, J. R. Swedlow, J. Vuong, and J. B. Procter, "Visualization of Biomedical Data," *Annual Review of Biomedical Data Science*, vol. 1, pp. 275–304, 2018. https://doi.org/10.1146/annurev-biodatasci-080917-013424.
3. Q. V. Nguyen, K. Zhang, and S. Simoff, "Unlocking the Complexity of Port Data With Visualization," *IEEE Transactions on Human-Machine Systems*, vol. 45, pp. 272–279, 2015. https://doi.org/10.1109/THMS.2014.2369375.
4. S. Boyd Davis, O. Vane, and F. Kräutli, "Can I Believe What I See? Data Visualization and Trust in the Humanities," *Interdisciplinary Science Reviews*, vol. 46, pp. 522–546. https://doi.org/10.1080/03080188.2021.1872874.
5. A. Chatzimparmpas, R. M. Martins, I. Jusufi, K. Kucher, F. Rossi, and A. Kerren, "The State of the Art in Enhancing Trust in Machine Learning Models with the Use of Visualizations," *Computer Graphics Forum*, vol. 39, pp. 713–756, 2020. https://doi.org/10.1111/cgf.14034.
6. Z. Qu, C. W. Lau, D. R. Catchpoole, S. Simoff, and Q. V. Nguyen, "Intelligent and Immersive Visual Analytics of Health Data," in *Advanced Computational Intelligence in Healthcare*, Maglogiannis, I., Brahnam, S., and Jain, L. C., Eds. Springer, 2020, pp. 29–44. https://doi.org/10.1007/978-3-662-61114-2_3.
7. A. Adadi and M. Berrada, "Peeking Inside the Black-Box: A Survey on Explainable Artificial Intelligence (XAI)," *IEEE Access*, vol. 6, pp. 52138–52160, 2018. https://doi.org/10.1109/ACCESS.2018.2870052.
8. E. Mayr, N. Hynek, S. Salisu, and F. Windhager, "Trust in Information Visualization," in *EuroVis Workshop on Trustworthy Visualization (TrustVis)*, 2019 of Conference. https://doi.org/10.2312/trvis.20191187.
9. J. Thomas and J. Kielman, "Challenges for Visual Analytics," *Information Visualization*, vol. 8, pp. 309–314, 2009.
10. J. Birkhäuer, J. Gaab, J. Kossowsky, S. Hasler, P. Krummenacher, C. Werner, and H. Gerger, "Trust in the Health Care Professional and Health Outcome: A Meta-Analysis," *PLOS One*, vol. 12, p. e0170988, 2017. https://doi.org/10.1371/journal.pone.0170988.

11. E. Toreini, M. Aitken, K. Coopamootoo, K. Elliott, C. G. Zelaya, and A. Van Moorsel, "The Relationship Between Trust in AI and Trustworthy Machine Learning Technologies," in *Proceedings of the 2020 Conference on Fairness, Accountability, and Transparency*, 2020, pp. 272–283.

12. Z. Qu, Y. Tegegne, S. J. Simoff, P. J. Kennedy, D. R. Catchpoole, and Q. V. Nguyen, "Enhancing Understandability of Omics Data with SHAP, Embedding Projections and Interactive Visualisations," in *Proceedings of Australasian Conference on Data Mining (AusDM 2022)*, Springer, 2022, pp. 58–72.

13. E. Beauxis-Aussalet, M. Behrisch, R. Borgo, D. H. Chau, C. Collins, D. Ebert, M. El-Assady, A. Endert, D. A. Keim, and J. Kohlhammer, "The Role of Interactive Visualization in Fostering Trust in Ai," *IEEE Computer Graphics and Applications*, vol. 41, pp. 7–12, 2021.

14. J. J. Caban and D. Gotz, "Visual Analytics in Healthcare – Opportunities and Research Challenges," *Journal of the American Medical Informatics Association*, vol. 22, pp. 260–262, 2015. https://doi.org/10.1093/jamia/ocv006.

15. G. S. Halford, R. Baker, J. E. McCredden, and J. D. Bain, "How Many Variables Can Humans Process?," *Psychological science*, vol. 16, pp. 70–76, 2005.

16. K. Börner, A. Bueckle, and M. Ginda, "Data Visualization Literacy: Definitions, Conceptual Frameworks, Exercises, and Assessments," *Proceedings of the National Academy of Sciences*, vol. 116, pp. 1857–1864, 2019. https://doi.org/10.1073/pnas.1807180116.

17. H.-K. Kong, Z. Liu, and K. Karahalios, "Trust and Recall of Information Across Varying Degrees of Title-visualization Misalignment," in *Proceedings of the 2019 CHI Conference on Human Factors in Computing Systems*, 2019, pp. 1–13.

18. K. Kim, J. V. Carlis, and D. F. Keefe, "Comparison Techniques Utilized in Spatial 3D and 4D Data Visualizations: A Survey and Future Directions," *Computers & Graphics*, vol. 67, pp. 138–147. https://doi.org/10.1016/j.cag.2017.05.005.

19. D. Ceneda, T. Gschwandtner, and S. Miksch, "A Review of Guidance Approaches in Visual Data Analysis: A Multifocal Perspective," *Computer Graphics Forum*, vol. 38, pp. 861–879, 2019. https://doi.org/10.1111/cgf.13730.

20. S. Coppers, J. V. D. Bergh, K. Luyten, K. Coninx, I. V. D. Lek-Ciudin, T. Vanallemeersch, and V. Vandeghinste, "Intellingo: An Intelligible Translation Environment," in *Proceedings of the 2018 CHI Conference on Human Factors in Computing Systems*, Montreal, ACM, 2018, p. 524. https://doi.org/10.1145/3173574.3174098.

21. A. Dasgupta, S. Burrows, K. Han, and P. J. Rasch, "Empirical Analysis of the Subjective Impressions and Objective Measures of Domain Scientists' Visual Analytic Judgments," in *Proceedings of the 2017 CHI Conference on Human Factors in Computing Systems*, ACM, 2017, pp. 1193–1204.

22. K. Kelton, K. R. Fleischmann, and W. A. Wallace, "Trust in Digital Information," *Journal of the American Society for Information Science and Technology*, vol. 59, pp. 363–374, 2008. https://doi.org/10.1002/asi.20722.

23. E. Mayr, N. Hynek, S. Salisu, and F. Windhager, "Trust in Information Visualization," in *TrustVis@ EuroVis*, 2019, pp. 25–29.
24. C. Hood and D. Heald, *Transparency: The Key to Better Governance?* vol. 135. Oxford: Oxford University Press for The British Academy, 2006.
25. F. L. Cook, L. R. Jacobs, and D. Kim, "Trusting What You Know: Information, Knowledge, and Confidence in Social Security," *The Journal of Politics*, vol. 72, pp. 397–412, 2010.
26. S. Joslyn and J. LeClerc, "Decisions with Uncertainty: The Glass Half Full," *Current Directions in Psychological Science*, vol. 22, pp. 308–315, 2013.
27. A. V. Pandey, A. Manivannan, O. Nov, M. Satterthwaite, and E. Bertini, "The Persuasive Power of Data Visualization," *IEEE Transactions on Visualization and Computer Graphics*, vol. 20, pp. 2211–2220, 2014. https://doi.org/10.1109/TVCG.2014.2346419.
28. L. Padilla, R. Fygenson, S. C. Castro, and E. Bertini, "Multiple Forecast Visualizations (MFVs): Trade-offs in Trust and Performance in Multiple COVID-19 Forecast Visualizations," *IEEE Transactions on Visualization and Computer Graphics*, vol. 29, pp. 12–22, 2022.
29. Z. Qu, Y. Zhou, Q. V. Nguyen, and D. R. Catchpoole, "Using Visualization to Illustrate Machine Learning Models for Genomic Data," in *Proceedings of the Australasian Computer Science Week Multiconference*, 2019, pp. 1–8.
30. C. Seifert, A. Aamir, A. Balagopalan, D. Jain, A. Sharma, S. Grottel, and S. Gumhold, "Visualizations of Deep Neural Networks in Computer Vision: A Survey," *Transparent Data Mining for Big and Small Data*, pp. 123–144, 2017.
31. W. Samek, T. Wiegand, and K.-R. Müller, "Explainable Artificial Intelligence: Understanding, Visualizing and Interpreting Deep Learning Models," *arXiv preprint arXiv:1708.08296*, 2017.
32. B. C. Kwon, H. Kim, E. Wall, J. Choo, H. Park, and A. Endert, "Axisketcher: Interactive Nonlinear Axis Mapping of Visualizations through User Drawings," *IEEE Transactions on Visualization and Computer Graphics*, vol. 23, pp. 221–230, 2016.
33. L. V. D. Maaten and G. Hinton, "Visualizing Data Using t-SNE," *Journal of Machine Learning Research*, vol. 9, pp. 2579–2605, 2008.
34. X. Zhao, Y. Wu, D. L. Lee, and W. Cui, "iforest: Interpreting Random Forests via Visual Analytics," *IEEE Transactions on Visualization and Computer Graphics*, vol. 25, pp. 407–416, 2018.
35. L. McInnes, J. Healy, and J. Melville, "UMAP: Uniform Manifold Approximation and Projection for Dimension Reduction," *arXiv:1802.03426 [stat.ML]*, 2018.
36. S. M. Lundberg and S.-I. Lee, "A Unified Approach to Interpreting Model Predictions," in *Proceedings of the 31st International Conference on Neural Information Processing Systems*, Long Beach, CA: Curran Associates Inc., 2017, pp. 4768–4777.
37. M. T. Ribeiro, S. Singh, and C. Guestrin, ""Why Should I Trust You?": Explaining the Predictions of Any Classifier," in *International Conference on Knowledge Discovery and Data Mining*, ed: ACM, 2016, pp. 1135–1144. https://doi.org/10.1145/2939672.2939778.

38. Q. A. Hathaway, S. M. Roth, M. V. Pinti, D. C. Sprando, A. Kunovac, A. J. Durr, C. C. Cook, G. K. Fink, T. B. Cheuvront, and J. H. Grossman, "Machine-learning to Stratify Diabetic Patients Using Novel Cardiac Biomarkers and Integrative Genomics," *Cardiovascular Diabetology*, vol. 18, pp. 1–16, 2019.

39. I. Palatnik de Sousa, M. Maria Bernardes Rebuzzi Vellasco, and E. Costa da Silva, "Local Interpretable Model-agnostic Explanations for Classification of Lymph Node Metastases," *Sensors*, vol. 19, p. 2969, 2019.

40. N. Thanh-Hai, T. B. Tran, A. C. Tran, and N. Thai-Nghe, "Feature Selection Using Local Interpretable Model-Agnostic Explanations on Metagenomic Data," in *International Conference on Future Data and Security Engineering*, 2020, pp. 340–357.

41. A. Orlenko and J. H. Moore, "A Comparison of Methods for Interpreting Random Forest Models of Genetic Association in the Presence of Non-additive Interactions," *BioData Mining*, vol. 14, p. 9. https://doi.org/10.1186/s13040-021-00243-0.

42. J. Hayakawa, T. Seki, Y. Kawazoe, and K. Ohe, "Pathway Importance by Graph Convolutional Network and Shapley Additive Explanations in Gene Expression Phenotype of Diffuse Large B-cell Lymphoma," *PLOS One*, vol. 17, p. e0269570, 2022.

Index